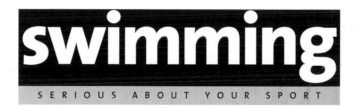

swimming

SERIOUS ABOUT YOUR SPORT

About the authors

Even breaking his neck, aged 16, in the pool could not put **Nic Newell** off swimming. Shortly afterwards he turned up at swimming carnival, took off his neck brace, won his race and calmly put the brace back on. A year later he was a three-time gold medallist in the Pacific School Games in Perth to add to his many achievements at state, regional and national level.

Dan Cross is the assistant National Age group coach at Guildford City High Performance Swimming Club. He has been coaching for almost 10 years after competing as a national standard swimmer for a number of years himself. He has coached age group, youth, senior and masters swimmers during his career, with many of the swimmers going on to achieve success at national level. He has coached at a number of different clubs and worked alongside many top international coaches. He has a degree in Sport and Exercise Science and a strong interest in sport science research.

Paul Cowcher has been working in the health and fitness industry since 2001 after a career as a professional dancer (musicals in West End and touring). When his dancing career was over he recognized there were many similarities between dancing and sports and science. He has trained as an advanced instructor (CYQ), Pilates mat work (More Fitness) and has over 10 other teaching qualifications in fitness and dance (ISTD.) He now works as a personal trainer.

Tommaso Bernabei is a television and non-fiction writer who graduated from the Metropolitan University of London. His experience in television led him to collaborate with Italian food shows, introducing him into the world of sports nutrition. He is currently the diet planner for an Italian swimming club and writing a book of sports nutrition recipes.

Photo Credits

iStockphoto.com and jacket, p159, Gabriella Fabbri – www.i-pix.it, www.sxc.hu. p12 Alx Sanchez – www.alxsanchez.com, www.sxc.hu. p12 Adsasd Asdsad – www.sxc.hu. p12 Luz Maria Espinoza – www.sxc.hu. p12 Sanja Gjenero – www.sxc.hu. p13 Marius Largu – www.lartekgrup.com www.sxc.hu. p15 Charles Thompson – www.cameraclash.com www.sxc.hu. p17 Galeria fotografii – rang.pl www.sxc.hu. p18 Iwan Beijes – www.beijesweb.nl www.sxc.hu. p18 Alex Bramwell – www.istockphoto.com/user_view.php www.sxc.hu. p18, p86 David Ritter – www.sxc.hu. p20 Richard Dudley – www.bluegumgraphics.com.au, www.sxc.hu. p20 Richard Dudley – www.bluegumgraphics.com.au www.sxc.hu. p21 Jocilyn Pope – www.sxc.hu. p21, p119 Pontus Edenberg – www.newsoffuture.com www.sxc.hu. p23 Lisa Ghaith – www.sxc.hu. p27 Albert Ip – www.sxc.hu. p33 Manfred Werner www.wikimedia.org. p37 Janusz Gawron – www.sxc.hu. p39 Cpl. Jasper Schwartz – www.wikimedia.org. p41 Manfred Werner – www.wikimedia.org. p86 Ramasamy Chidambaram – www.studiosrishti.com, www.sxc.hu. p86 Cienpies Design – www.cienpies.net, www.sxc.hu. p119 Jonathan Ruchti, Switzerland – www.sxc.hu. p119 Lukas – www.blogonade.de – www.sxc.hu. p119 Jonathan Ruchti, Switzerland – www.sxc.hu. p122 Pedro Simao – www.editae.com.br, www.sxc.hu. p122 Rob Owen-Wahl – www.LockStockPhotography.com, www.sxc.hu. p122 Agata Urbaniak – www.xero.prv.pl, www.sxc.hu. p126 Ove Tøpfer – www.pixelmaster.no, www.sxc.hu. p126 Ove Tøpfer – www.pixelmaster.no, www.sxc.hu. p126 Emre Nacigil – www.atolyekusadasi.com, www.sxc.hu. p130 Anna H-G – www.sxc.hu. p130 Alaa Hamed – users2.titanichost.com/alaasafei, www.sxc.hu. p130 Gunnar Brink – www.sxc.hu. p137 Rob Owen-Wahl – www.LockStockPhotography.com, www.sxc.hu. p138 Kliverap – www.sxc.hu. p138 Brandon Kettle – www.sxc.hu. p138 Johan Bolhuis – www.natuurarts.nl, www.sxc.hu. p139 Pedro Simao – www.editae.com.br, www.sxc.hu. p139 Michael Grunow – www.sxc.hu. p139 Monika M – www.sxc.hu. p140 Gerhard Taatgen jr. – www.taatgen-fotografie.nl, www.sxc.hu. p140 Neil Gould – http://gallery.gouldnet.net, www.sxc.hu. p140 Meekes – www.sxc.hu. p141 Lukas – www.blogonade.de – www.sxc.hu. p141 Matteo Canessa – www.sxc.hu. p141 Chris Greene – www.sxc.hu. p142 Aschaeffer – www.sxc.hu. p142 Brandon W. Mosley – http://www.manjidesigns.com, www.sxc.hu. p142 Steph P – www.sxc.hu. p143 Lavinia Marin – www.sxc.hu. p143 Luca Baroncini – www.cggallery.it, www.sxc.hu. p143 hde2003 – www.sxc.hu. p159 Lotus Head – www.pixelpusher.co.za, www.sxc.hu. p159 Manfred Werner www.wikimedia.org. Notepad graphic Davide Guglielmo – www.broken-arts.com, www.sxc.hu.

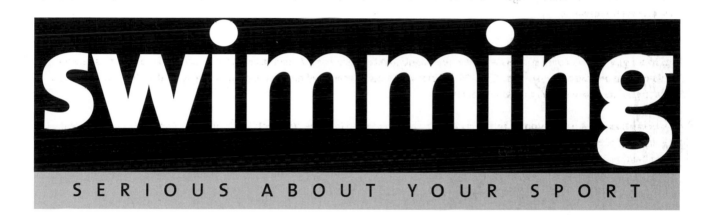

swimming

SERIOUS ABOUT YOUR SPORT

Nic Newell, Dan Cross, Paul Cowcher and Tommaso Bernabei

Additional writing: Adam Hathaway and Remmert Wielinga

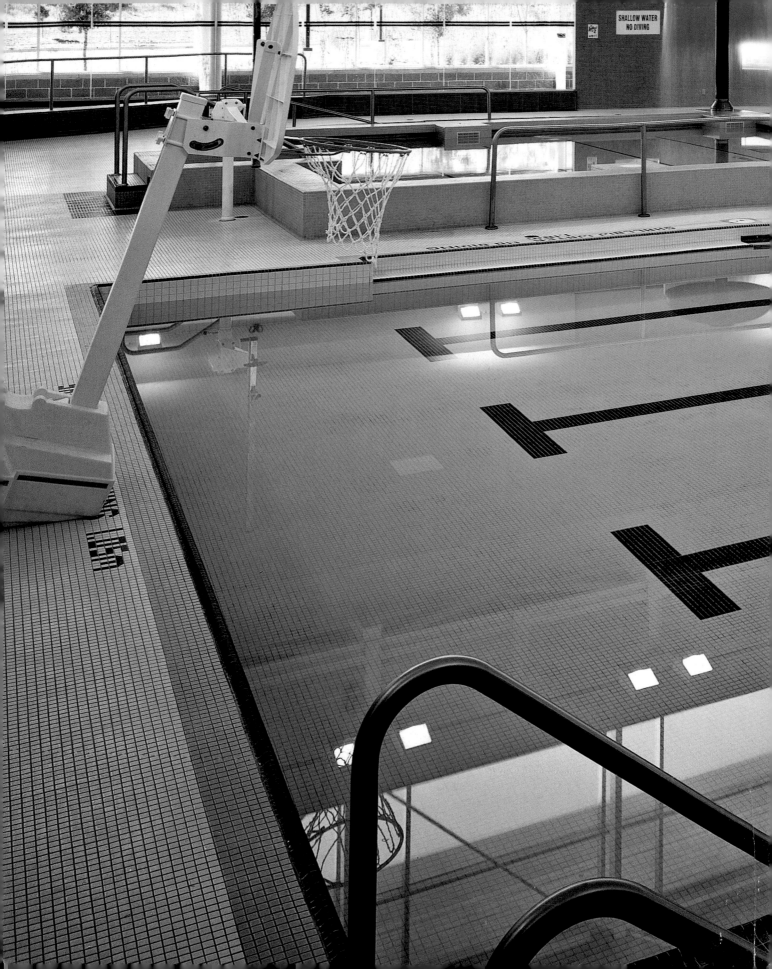

SHALLOW WATER
NO DIVING

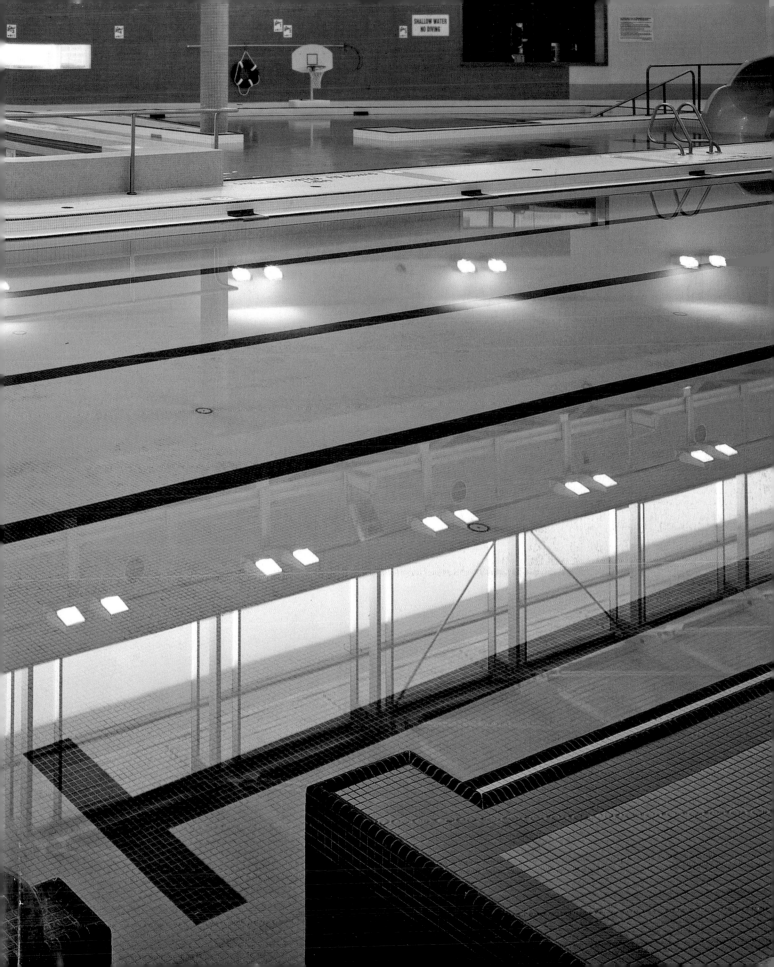

Contents

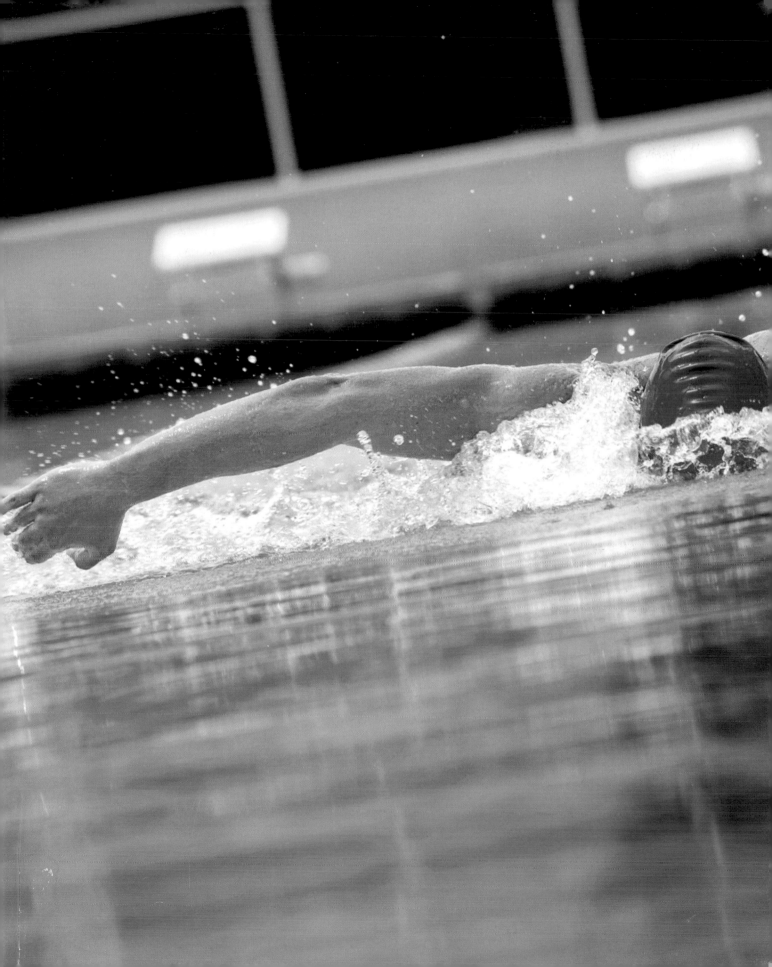

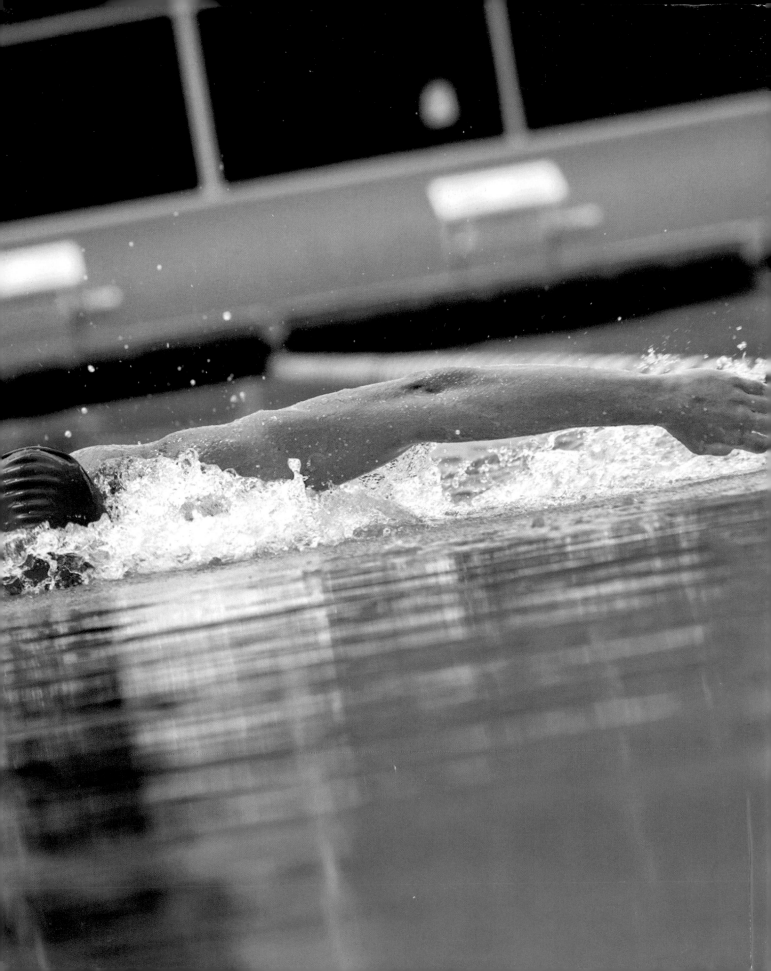

Introduction

Diving into the water, to prepare for my backstroke leg, ahead of the final of the 4x100m medley relay at the Pacific School Games in Perth in 1997 my thoughts kept going back to the hours and hours of training I had put in just to get there.

By the age of 17 I had virtually swum enough lengths of the training pool to get me from Sydney, where I learned to swim aged three, to the west coast of Australia.

Why swimming? My attempts to emulate Wally Lewis on the rugby pitch had come to nothing and I was no Shane Warne with a cricket ball so when a local coach saw something to work on in the pool my mind was made up. It is relatively cheap, keeps you fit and, at times, can be a sociable sport when you meet for inter-club races and carnivals.

On the flip side it can be lonely. I even learnt to have conversations with friends while I was ploughing up and down the pool, in training in Sydney, that was named after John Devitt, who won gold at the 1960 Olympic Games in Rome in the 100 metres freestyle. Moving onto Guildford Swimming Pool, aged 13, to be trained under David Wick with McCredie Park Swimming Club I moved up another notch.

Although I never made it to Devitt's standard, and have never had a pool named after me, I still had to give up quite a lot to get to the Pacific Games. Arriving at the pool at dawn before school, nine training sessions in the water every week before and after lessons, a couple of gym sessions and a Sunday meet every other week meant that my teenage years were not typical. No burgers or ribs for a week leading up to a race... agony for a growing boy... and I was training so much I didn't take one lunch box to school: I was so hungry I took four...

This book is for swimmers who want to aim that little bit higher. You don't have to make yourself a slave to the sport like I did but by adhering to a few principles in training, in and out of the pool, and maintaining some good lifestyle habits you will soon knock seconds off your time and do yourself some good in the process.

Not everyone can be a Mark Spitz or an Ian Thorpe but everyone can be better at swimming. You can't get a bad bounce of the ball, won't get beaten by a poor refereeing decision and no-one else can affect your performance. It is the ultimate no-excuses sport.

Clutching the wall at the start of the final, with swimmers from all over the world surrounding me, I thought about all of that. All those sacrifices for a few minutes in the pool and a few paragraphs in the local paper. Was it worth it?

In a word yes.

I have got a gold medal somewhere in the attic that says it was worth it. It might not be the same as Devitt's but it means a lot to me. Maybe you can get one too.

Nic Newell
June 2010

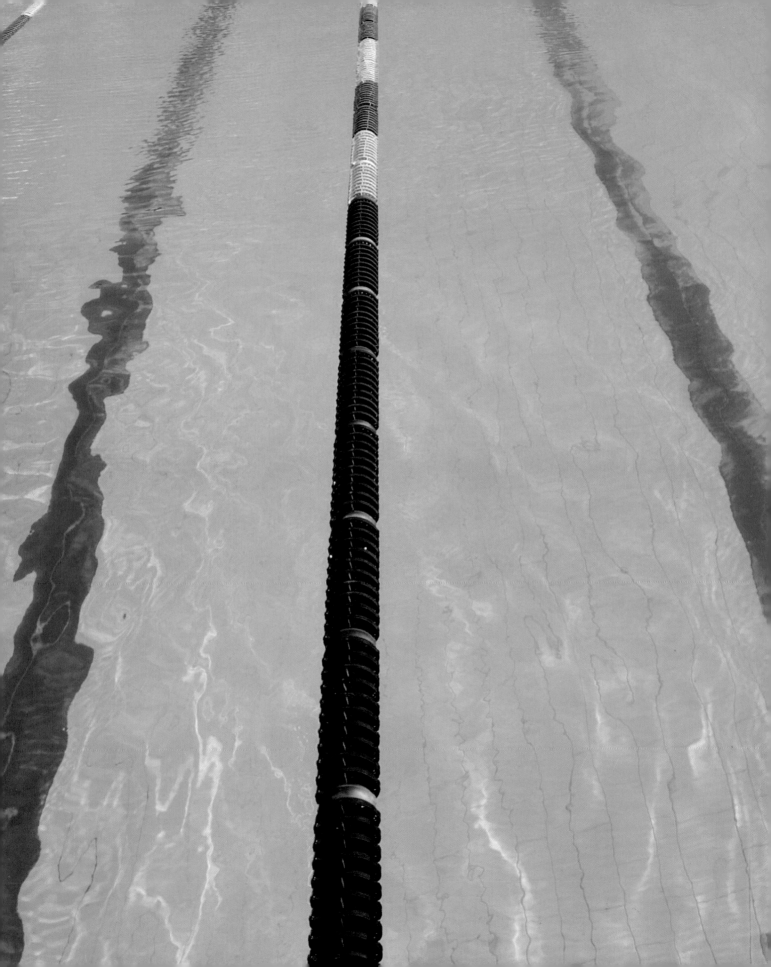

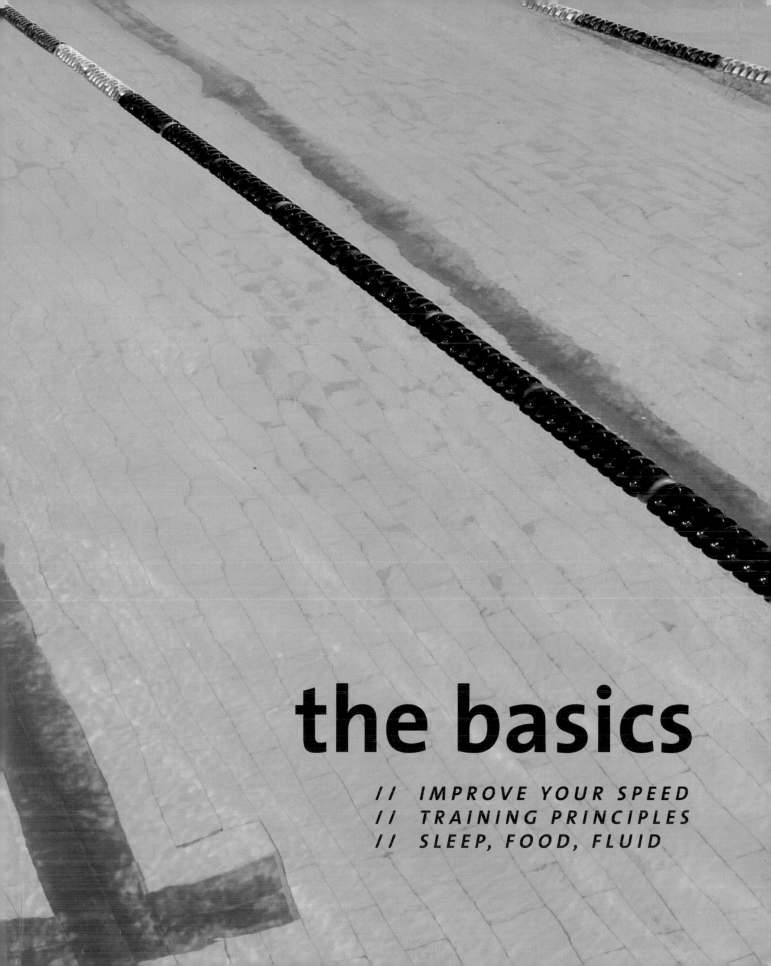

the basics

// IMPROVE YOUR SPEED
// TRAINING PRINCIPLES
// SLEEP, FOOD, FLUID

Getting started

So you enjoy swimming and have decided you want to get serious about your training in the pool, but you are not sure where to start? First, you need to ask yourself honestly: "Am I physically capable of upping my game or should I stay as a social swimmer? Do I have enough time on my hands to commit to an intensive programme that will allow me to become a stronger and faster swimmer."

If you are unsure about any aspects of your health you should always check with a doctor before embarking on a new fitness programme to make sure you are physically fit for the challenge. You also have to consider work and family commitments and put every-thing into balance. It's certainly not impossible to have young children, a demanding job and still train hard for swimming but it will require a lot of planning and determination.

Once you have the green light to go for it you then need to decide what you are training for and why? Maybe you want to improve your distance swimming or maybe it's your sprint speed you want to fine-tune. Your goal maybe to compete in your first swimming race or it maybe to improve the standard of your swimming for a triathlon you are entering.

It doesn't matter if you are trying to compete at the highest level or if you are competing against yourself, by making sure you are in the right shape to get started you will make the training far more effective and more enjoyable. Don't expect to become a national champion in a couple of months if you have only just learnt to swim or you aren't physically ready for it. You need to choose realistic goals and have a realistic time scale for when you want to reach the goals. Start by

jotting down what you want out of your swimming and what your goals are; this will help you visualize where you are going and help to keep you focused as your training gets more intense.

Developing a long-term goal will help you decide on what type of training is best for you and how you can get the most out of your training plan. You may have a target competition to train for or you might simply want to swim 50m or 1500m in a new personal best time.

By setting targets and goals you can focus on what you want to achieve and help keep motivation levels high while you are training. Good luck! Training can be hard work and at times lonely, but the rewards can be huge. Don't be deterred, just keep your eye on the end results.

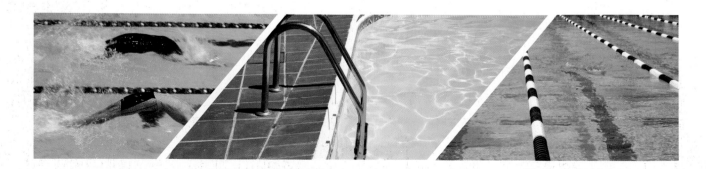

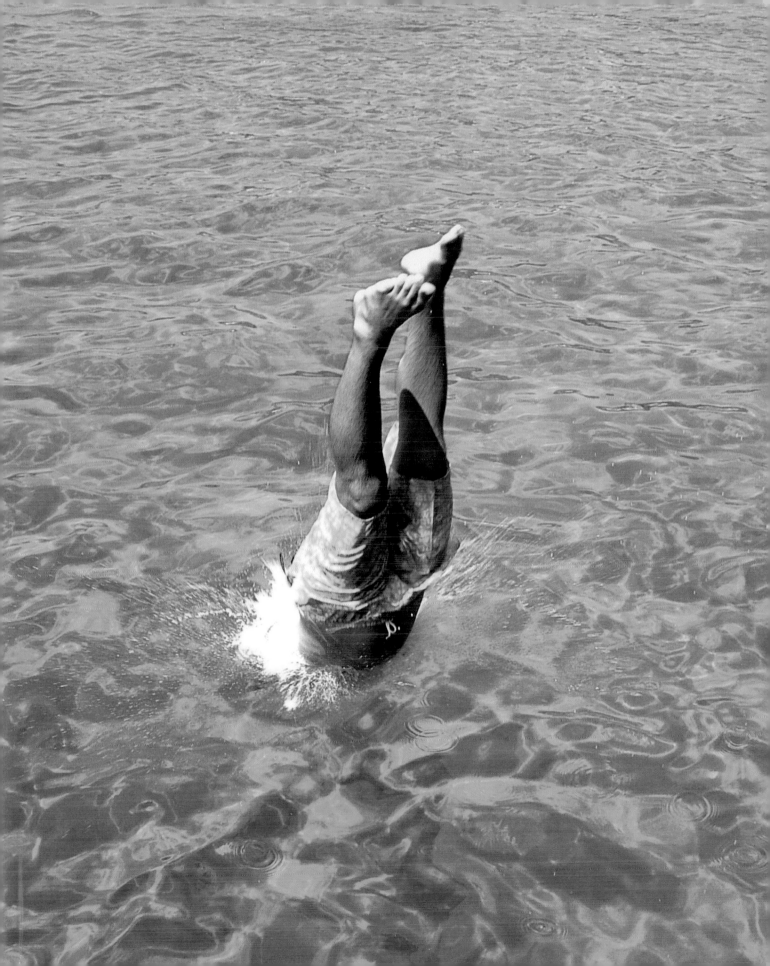

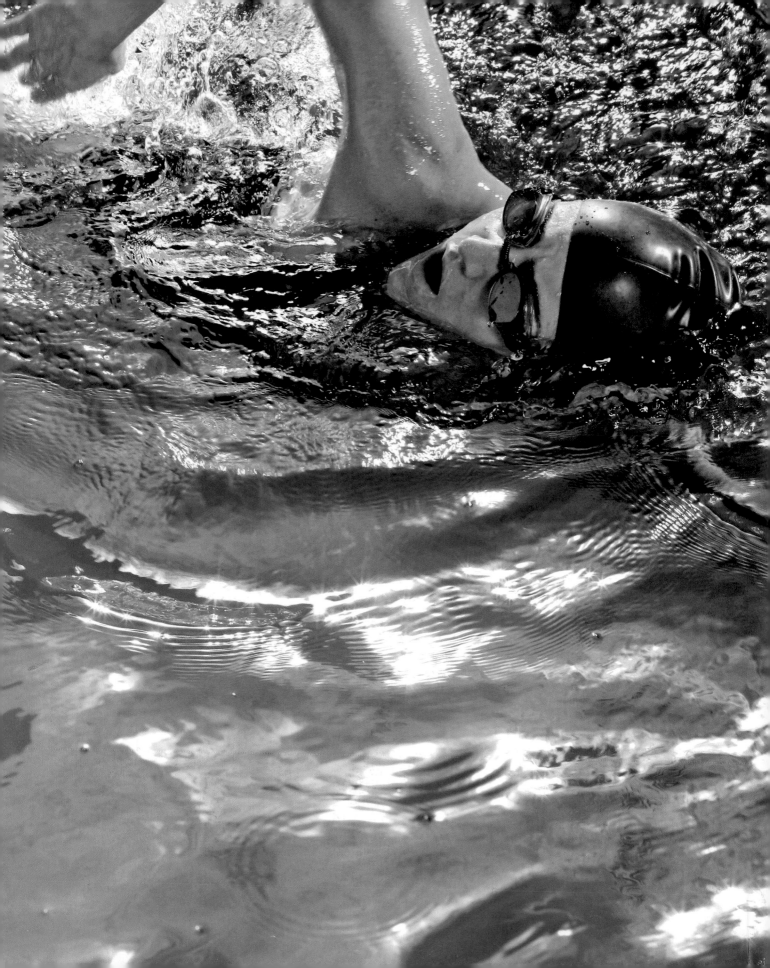

Preparing to improve your speed

There are many factors involved in improving swimming speed and these are: technique, fitness levels, nutrition, rest and the suitability of your training.

Technique will play a large part in swimming faster. If you can improve your technique it will help improve the efficiency of your stroke and conserve energy. An inefficient stroke will use a lot of wasted energy that does nothing to improve speed. The more efficient your stroke is the more energy you are conserving to be used later in the race or the more that is being transferred into swimming at a faster pace.

It sounds simple enough but many people, in many sports, continue to expend unnecessary energy that is quite simply getting them nowhere fast. Improve your technique and concentrate on maintaining that technique even when tired because

it's the surest way you have of improving your speed.

When deciding on a training plan you should assess your current level of fitness to ensure that the training goals you set yourself are not only realistic but also safe for your current fitness levels. If your fitness levels are low then don't set yourself too great a target as this will mean you over-train and injure yourself. You can do nothing when injured except get frustrated.

Equally you need to choose a plan that will require you to be constantly challenging yourself, so make sure your plan is always pushing your fitness levels. Don't let your body get used to its level of training; keep pushing it upwards. But, very importantly, when you are constantly pushing yourself in training you must make time for rest and recovery. You need to allow time for your body to recover and allow

for adaptations to occur as well as allowing your energy stores to be replaced so you are ready for your next training session.

The fitter you are the less time it will take for your body to recover. As you start to adapt to the training you will be able to start doing more training and increase the duration of the sessions but you will still need to make plenty of time for rest and recovery.

Nutrition can play an important role in your training. Maintaining energy and hydration levels before, during and after training (and in competition) will improve your level of performance and help you maintain focus. Poor nutrition can leave you feeling tired before and during training and can also slow down your recovery from intense training as well as leaving you more susceptible to illness and injury.

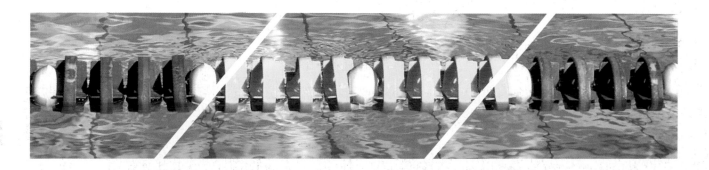

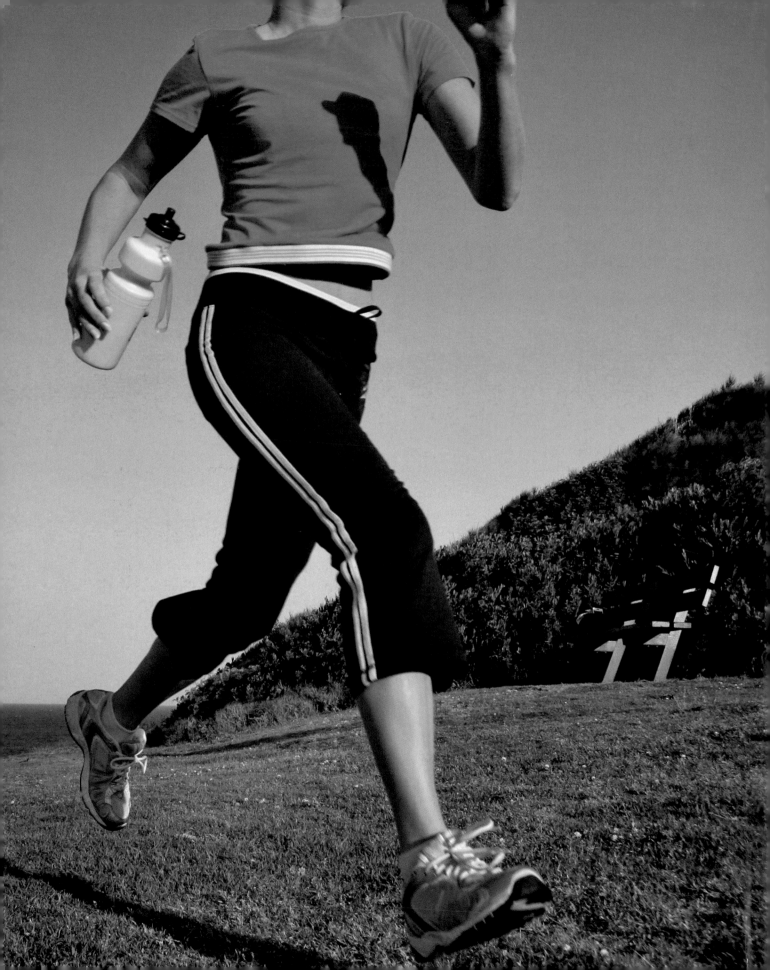

The principles of training

The **SPORT** principles of training are aimed at helping you understand the training process and allowing you to plan your training so you see a steady upward progression in results.

Specificity – making sure your training is specific to what you are hoping to achieve. Simply put, don't spend all your time doing sprint training sets if you want to improve your long-distance swimming!

Progression – the body adapts to increased training loads and this will result in improved fitness levels and competitive performance.

Overload – training at a level that will push you. If you are always training at the same intensity and at the same speed you will not see the progression you would hope for. You need to be constantly overloading your muscles and cardio respiratory system to improve your strength and fitness level.

Reversibility – if you don't train or you decrease your intensity then you will see your fitness levels drop and as a consequence so will your overall performance. If you are unwell and are unable to train for an extended period then you will notice a reduced performance level when you start training again.

Tedium – keeping the training interesting. If you find yourself getting bored then you are less likely to want to train and your motivation levels will automatically drop, which can lead to a reduced effort level and even the likelihood of skipping training sessions. This will lead to Reversibility occurring.

When you start to plan your training programme you can use the FITT principles to work towards SPORT. For instance, to make sure that the SPORT principles of Progression and Overload are always occurring you can increase the Frequency of your training sessions, the Intensity of each session or the Time you spend training. To stop Reversibility occurring rapidly you reduce Intensity if feeling sick. To avoid the SPORT principle of Tedium you can change the Type of training methods you are using. It is advisable that you only change one aspect of the training at a time rather than changing everything otherwise it can be too much for your body and may lead to an injury occurring.

Frequency – how often you train

Intensity – intensity you train at

Time – how long you train for

Type – which training methods you are using

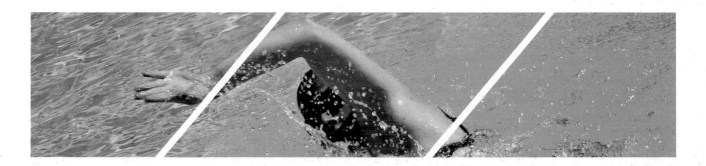

Getting ready to train

Before you jump into the water and swim those first metres it is important that your body and your mind are ready to train. Don't fall into the trap of thinking you can simply warm-up during training, even if it is going to be a relatively long session. Your body needs to be prepared and warned what it is going to be expected to do in the coming session and thanks to five to 10 minutes warming up your training sessions will start and run much more smoothly (as will your body).

Everyone has busy schedules and pressing commitments on their time, but now you have made the effort to come to training don't ruin what could be a good session by trying to save a few minutes by skipping the warming up part of training. In fact, if you really must cut down on your time then you should rather choose to reduce your training session than cut out your warm-up. Make it part of your routine, not something to get out of the way before you start the 'real training'.

Some basic body movement exercises will help loosen the muscles and prepare them for the training that is to follow (see Fitness & Training on pages 75-81). The idea of these stretches are to loosen the joints that you are about to use in training without putting any resistance on the joint and to help increase the blood flow around the muscles that support the joint. This will help to reduce the chance of injury occurring. These minutes on the side of the pool preparing your muscles should become an important part of every training session you do.

Mentally, whatever else is going on in your life, try to spend a few minutes thinking of your upcoming session, whether this is in the car on the way to training or even while you are getting changed. Shut out your problems at work and at home for a short time. Remind yourself why you are training and remind yourself of the benefits you have already gained from previous sessions. Try to think through the session ahead and focus on getting as much out of it as possible, in terms of achievement, and, of course, enjoyment. Then get started and enjoy your training!

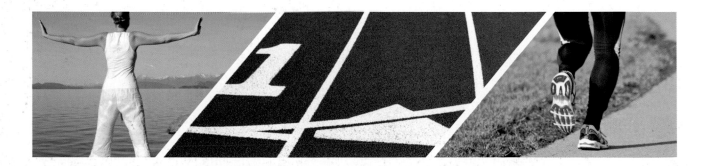

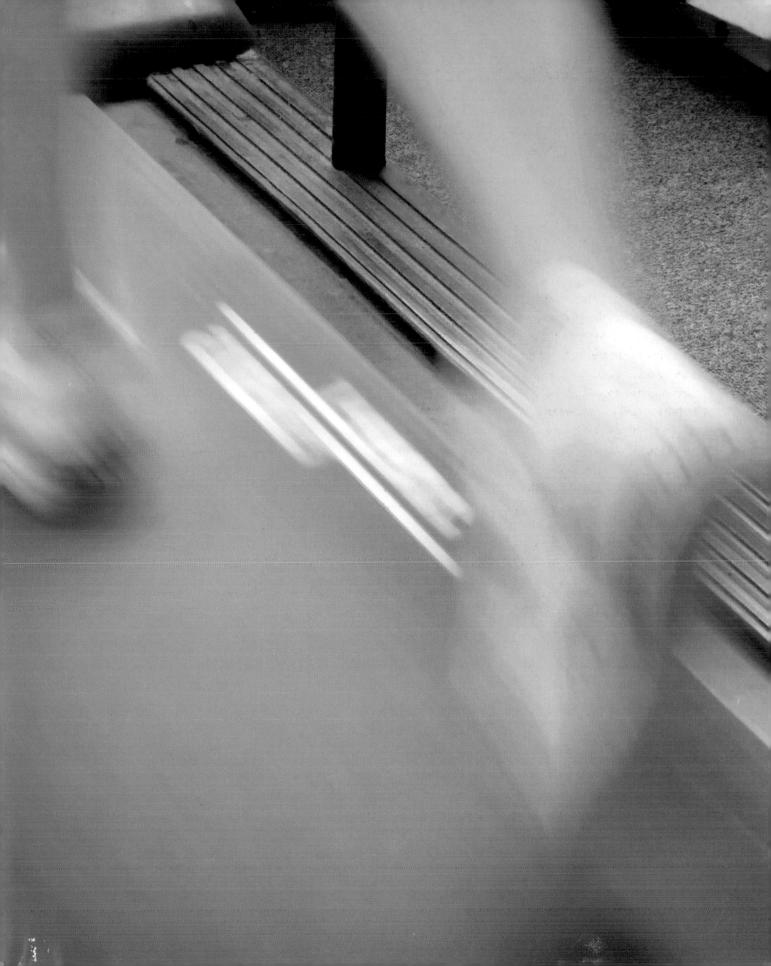

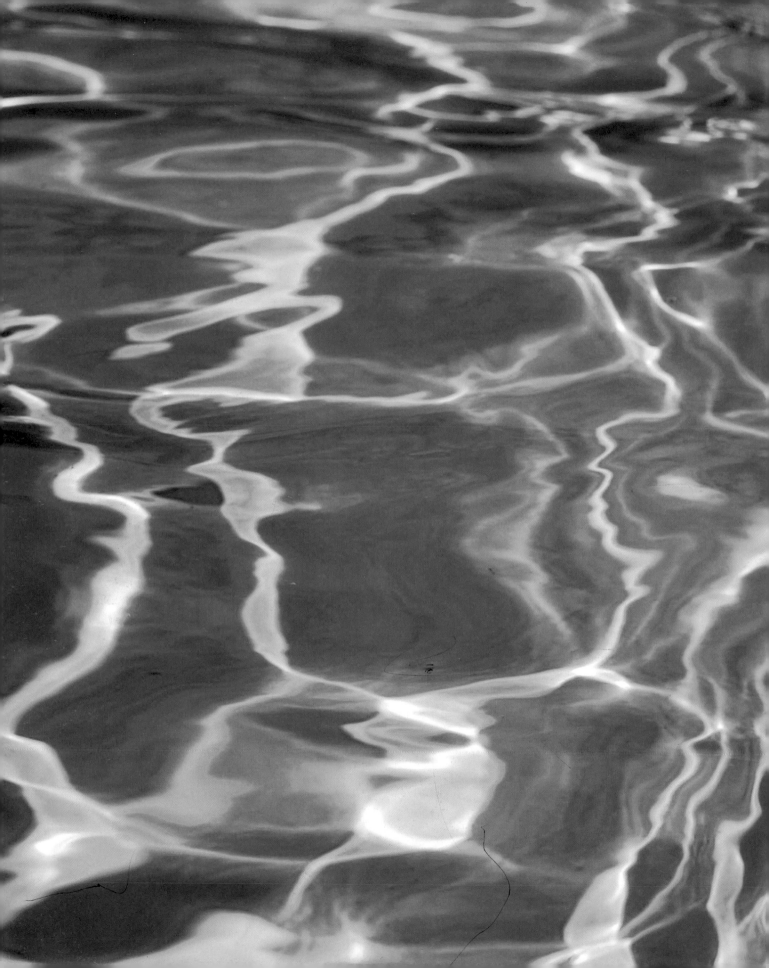

Sleep, food and fluid

Getting your work-to-rest ratio right is crucial, as an imbalance will lead to overtraining, which may result in a decreased performance in training and racing, as well as an increased chance of injury. Put simply: rest is as important as the training itself. As you get fitter you will be able to train longer as long as you keep getting quality rest.

- Set a schedule: be strict in your sleep regime. Sleep and wake at the same time every day including weekends and try to get at least eight hours of rest. Disrupting this schedule may lead to insomnia. 'Catching up' by sleeping extra on weekends makes it harder to wake up early on Monday morning because it re-sets your sleep cycles.

- Exercise: daily exercise will help you sleep, although a workout too close to your bedtime may disrupt your sleep. For maximum benefit try to get your exercise about five to six hours before going to bed.

- Avoid caffeine, nicotine, and alcohol. Don't take these stimulants close to your bedtime. Remember there is caffeine in coffee, chocolate, soft drinks, non-herbal teas, diet drugs and some pain relievers. Don't smoke a cigarette before going to bed as nicotine goes straight to the sleep centres of your brain and will result in a bad night's rest. Alcohol can decrease the time required to fall asleep. However, too much alcohol consumed within an hour of bedtime will deprive you of deep sleep and REM sleep (the sleep that rejuvenates your body the best) and it will keep you in the lighter stages of sleep.

- Relax before bed: reading, listening to music, having sex, taking a warm bath, can all make it easier to fall asleep. You can train yourself to associate certain activities with sleep and make them part of your bedtime ritual. If you can't get to sleep, don't just lie in bed – relax and do something else (like the previously mentioned activities) until you feel tired.

- Control your room temperature: make sure that you sleep in a room that is cool – 18-19 °C (64-66 °F) with 65 per cent of humidity is ideal – as well as dark and quiet.

So train hard and rest well. Nutrition can help supplement your training by giving you the right balance of energy to train and the proteins, vitamins and minerals to help you recover. If you are not getting the right levels of carbohydrates, proteins, fats and vitamins you will quickly feel tired in training and will fail to recover properly, which can lead to fatigue and maybe illness and injury. Hydration is critical, as the body has to be topped up to perform at its peak. Even a one per cent drop in hydration levels will impair your performance. Get used to taking on fluids.

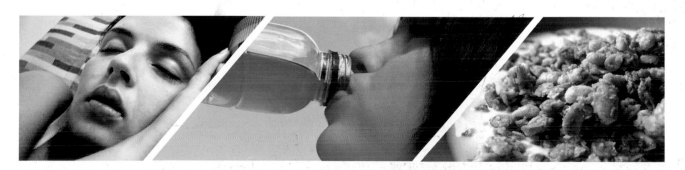

Equipment

That'll be a swimming costume and some water then. It can be as simple as that but using the right equipment can make training a lot more effective and enjoyable and it also allows for you to add variety to each training session. The basics are a suitable swimming costume, a pair of goggles, a swimming cap and a drinks bottle. Some people don't like swimming caps but it will make it easier to swim especially if you have long hair as it keeps the hair out of your face when you are turning your head to breathe.

Other pieces of training equipment include a kick board and a pull buoy. These items allow you to isolate areas of each stroke and work them on their own. You can use a kick board to work on your leg kick – you could be either trying to perfect technique or trying to improve leg-kick speed. A pull buoy is used to work on the arm-stroke technique. Pull sets are also used to help improve stroke technique as well as your stroke efficiency. By isolating parts of the stroke you can make your sets more challenging as you are trying to propel yourself through the water with only half the usual power.

If you want to make pull sets even more challenging you can wear hand paddles; these will allow you to put greater pressure on the water and therefore greater pressure on the arm and shoulders. Paddles should only be worn if you are already achieving good stroke technique and you need to take your pull sets to the next level. You must also make sure that you build your pull sets up gradually to avoid any shoulder injuries. When using paddles you should select the right paddles for your experience level as they come in different shapes and sizes, with the bigger paddles putting more pressure on the stroke.

A pair of fins can be used for kick sets as well as being used for full-stroke swims. Wearing fins can make swimming full-stroke swims easier, which means you are able to focus on stroke technique. They can also make certain strokes such as butterfly easier so you are able to cover more distance and work on your technique.

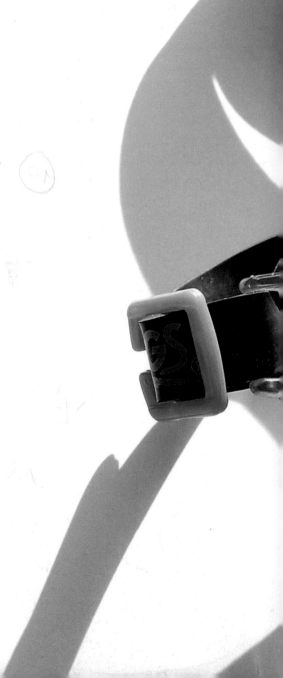

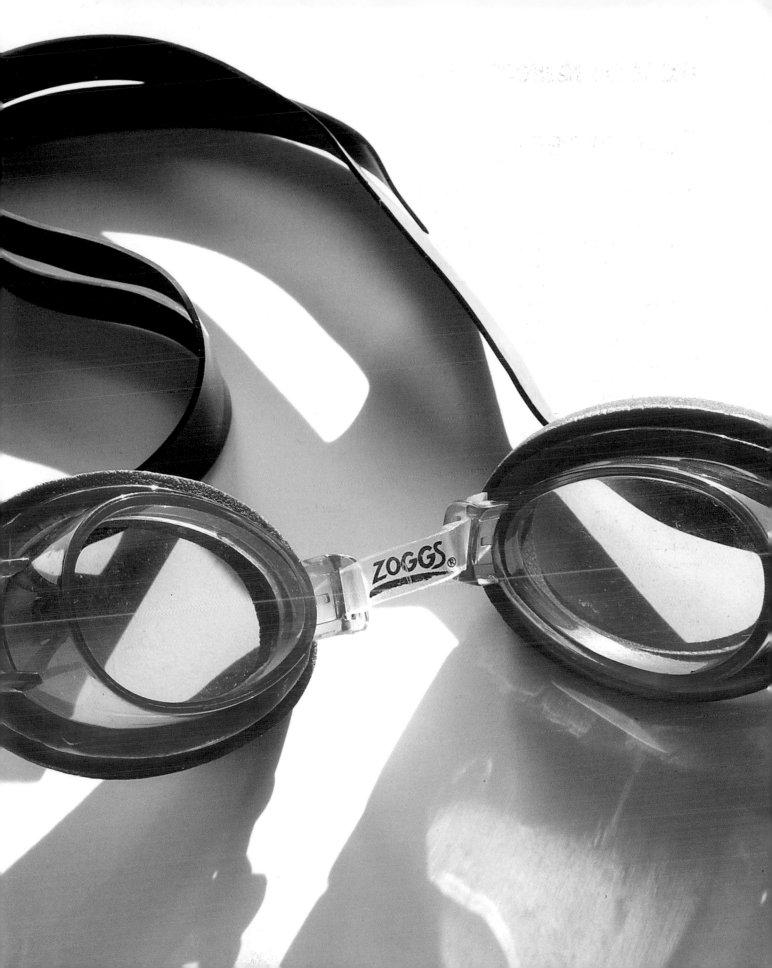

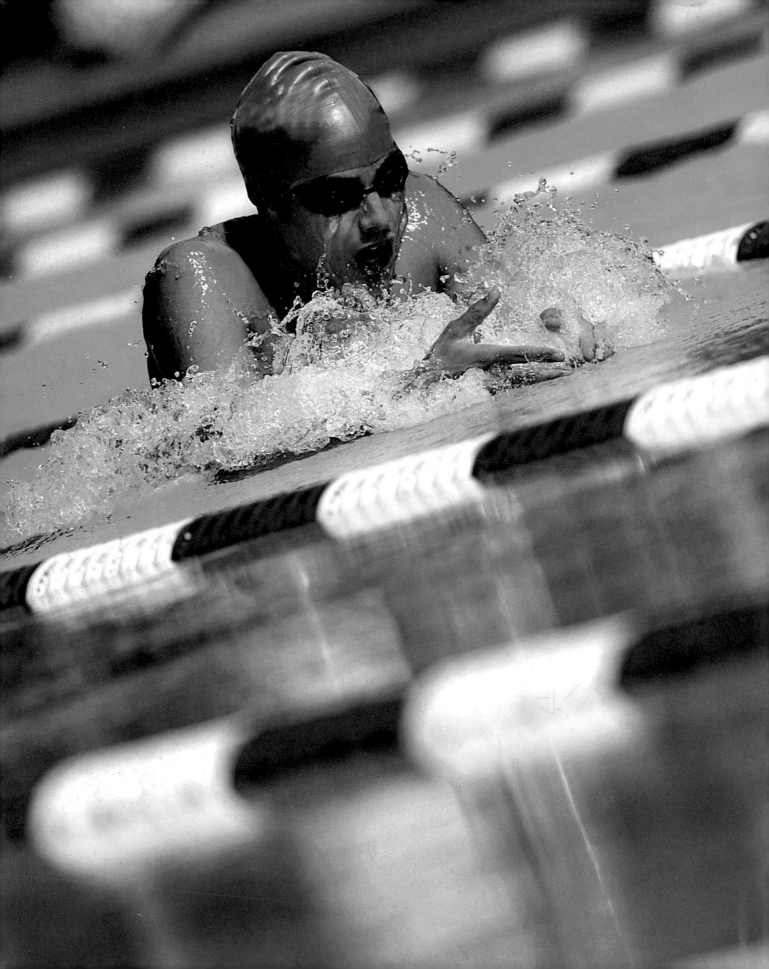

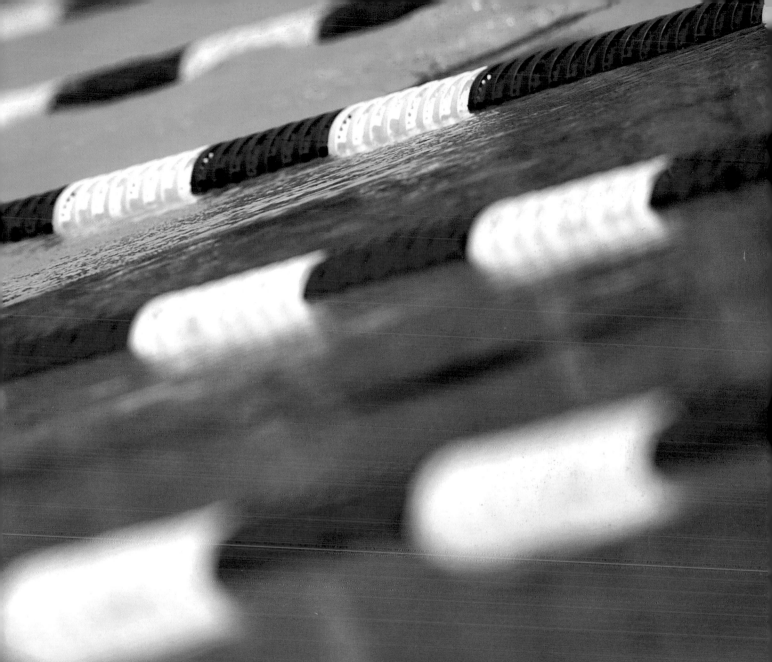

technique
& tactics

// SHARPER // SMARTER // MORE EFFICIENT

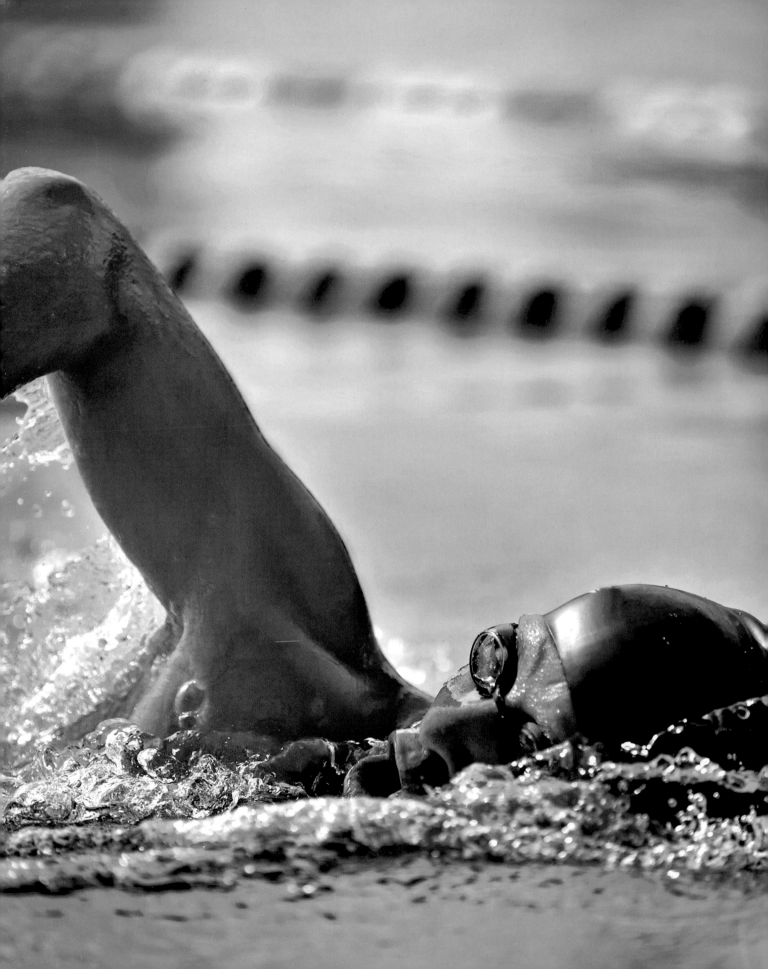

The basics

Everyone enjoys time in the water but how many of us could improve our times without hardly any effort at all? The answer is... virtually everyone. With a few basic technical hints and tips you can shave seconds off your personal best whether your target is a first race for your club or a regional championship final. It is never too late to learn and never too late to fine-tune your technique.

Many non-professional swimmers plough up and down the lanes of their local pool with little knowledge of the basics that could help them get better and swim faster. If you just want a few minutes exercise a couple of times a week, then that maybe is fine, but if you are looking to take that extra step in this sport then it is vital to look at how your body works in the pool and see where its efficiency can

be improved. You will see the results on the clock very quickly.

Along the way it will make your swimming even more enjoyable. Having the physique of a top-class athlete is not enough to get better but a little understanding of the mechanics of the various strokes can go a long way to improving your performance in the water. And the good news is, it is not rocket science – most of the principles are straightforward common sense.

The majority of the aspects of technique are about making the stroke more efficient, which in turn makes them less tiring, which in turn means you can go faster for longer without spending hundreds of hours pumping iron in the gym. Swimming is also the only sport where virtually every muscle group in the body is employed at the same

time, adding to the overall benefit. You don't have to work each group one at a time, like you do in the gym, they are all being exercised simultaneously.

The four strokes: backstroke, breaststroke, butterfly and freestyle employ many of the same principles such as using arms and legs in unison, making maximum use of your hands and feet to move you more quickly through the water and maintaining a streamlined position to decrease your resistance in the water. The strokes are complementary, but working on one will help you improve another as you utilise previously unused muscles. Most people have a preference for one or the other of the strokes but can bring their weaker strokes up to speed with the basic hints we have outlined on the next few pages.

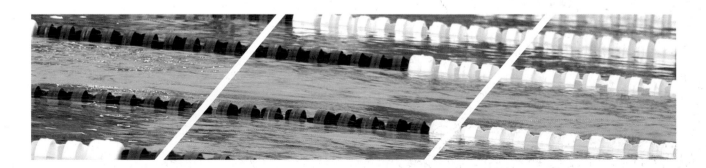

Backstroke

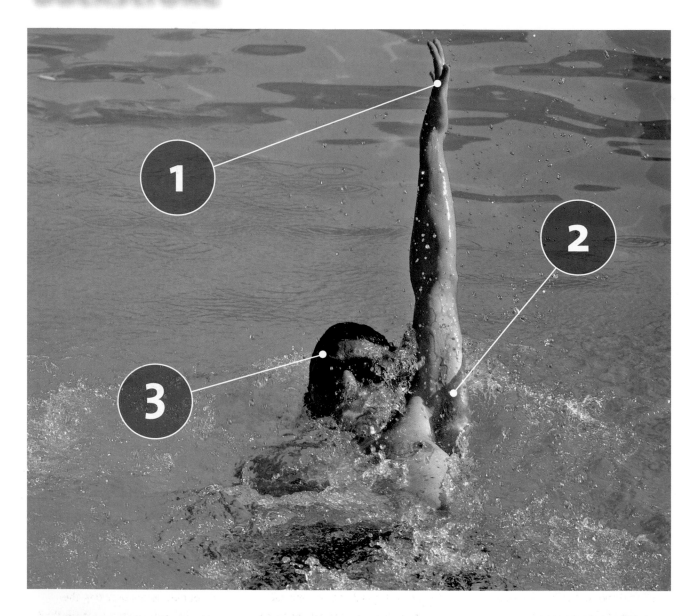

1 Your thumb should leave the water first; your little finger enters first. This maximises shoulder turn and power.

2 Keep your shoulders and chest above the water with your hips just beneath the surface.

3 It is vital to keep your head as still as possible for good balance.

As with all strokes, getting your body position right in the water is important in making the whole process as efficient as possible. With backstroke you should be trying to get the whole of your body up near the top of the water to reduce the resistance.

Your head needs to be sat in the water with your eyes looking at the ceiling and your ears just at the surface. Keeping your head still is important, because lifting or moving your head at any stage will alter your body position and add resistance to the body.

Your shoulders and chest should be sat clear of the surface with your hips ever so slightly submerged. Your shoulders will roll around the long axis as each arm stroke is performed. As one hand enters the water, the opposite shoulder will rotate out of the water to reduce water resistance and allow a deeper catch on the stroke due to increased range of motion.

Your head should be kept perfectly still and looking up as your shoulders rotate to help balance the rest of the body in the water. Your hips should also rotate at the same time as your shoulders – this will help improve your body's stream-lined position in the water.

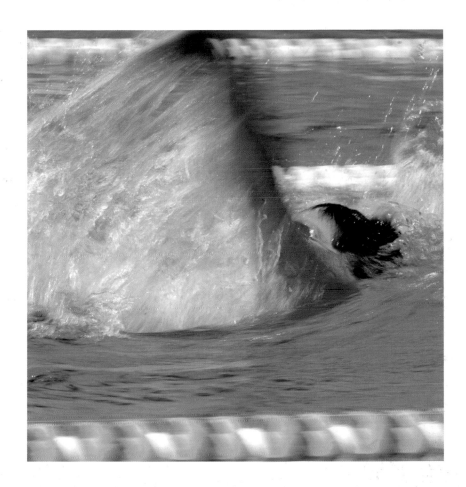

Leg Kick

Like freestyle, the backstroke stroke uses an alternating leg kick, which needs to be constant to maintain your body position in the water. A six-beat leg kick is the preferred kicking pattern, which means three kicks per arm stroke and six kicks per arm cycle.

Your legs should be kept long, and you should flex only a small amount from the knee as the kick needs to come from the hip. As your knee kicks up towards the surface your legs should straighten as the toe just breaks the surface. At no point should your knee break the surface; if your knees are breaking the surface of the water it means that your legs are not straight enough on the upwards phase of your kick.

Your toe needs to be turned just inwards to ensure you are getting enough power from each kick; poor ankle flexibility will also reduce the power from each kick and this will make it a less efficient stroke.

Arms

The recovery phase of the stroke is when your arm is out of the water. At this stage your arm should be straight and be kept as close to your body's central line as possible.

When your arm leaves the water your thumb should exit first and as your arm is recovering your hand should be rotated so that the little finger can enter first – this

✓ Do keep a continuous arm stroke. One arm in, one arm out.

✗ Don't move your head around – it reduces balance.

✓ Do keep your shoulder and chest above the water.

✗ Don't let your hips go above the surface.

✓ Rotate your hips simultaneously with your shoulders.

✗ Don't flex your knee much in the kick – the power should come from your hips.

✓ Keep a regular breathing cycle – it helps prevent fatigue.

✗ Don't use the flutter kick apart from underwater at the start and turns.

helps with the rotation of your shoulder. As your arm enters the water your elbow will be pointing down with your arms straight and wrist extended. At this point you are trying to catch the water before starting with the propulsion phase.

To start the catch you need to be pressing on the water with your hand angled down and slightly out. At this point your opposite shoulder will be rotating out of the water to allow you to propel quicker through the water and give you an increased range of shoulder motion. After the initial catch and start of the propulsion phase your hand should start to angle towards your feet as your elbow bends and points towards the bottom of the pool.

Your arm must continue sweeping until it is directly under your shoulder where it is almost at its deepest point. It should then start to sweep towards your hips and should vigorously move back towards the surface as your arm straightens and prepares to exit the water below your hip. It is important that your hand is always pressing on the water, palm first on the pull stroke, as that will ensure your thumb exits the water first and

you are not slipping water, which reduces your speed.

Breathing

Breathing will occur when needed on backstroke as your head is always above water, which is unlike the other strokes where you are restricted. Breathing should be kept regular and steady and will increase as the workload increases.

Timing

As well as maintaining the six-beat leg kick during every arm cycle it is important you always keep your arm strokes continuous. While one arm is recovering over the water your other arm should be propelling through the water. By maintaining a continuous stroke rate you will be helping to keep your body at the surface of the water where it has the least resistance.

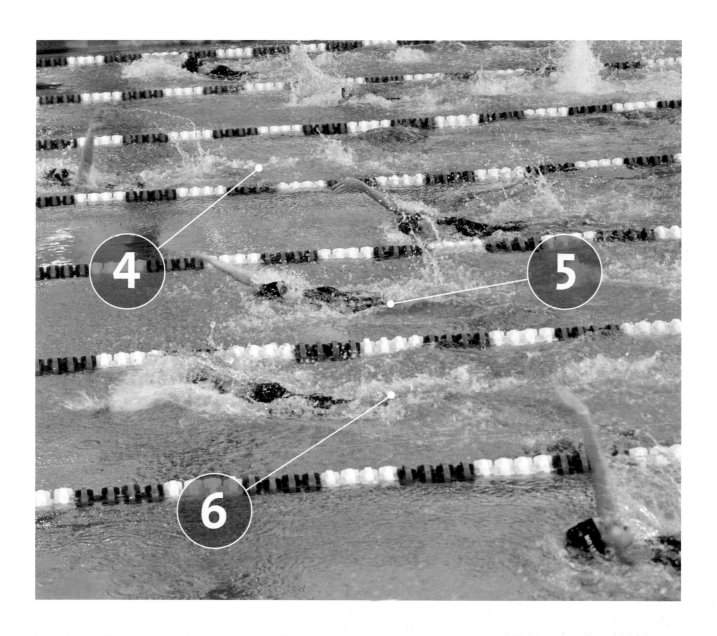

4 Your legs should kick alternately in the reverse of a freestyle kick.

5 Kick your legs from the hips to give yourself a bigger lever to work in the water.

6 To maintain a streamlined position your knees should not come above the surface.

Breaststroke

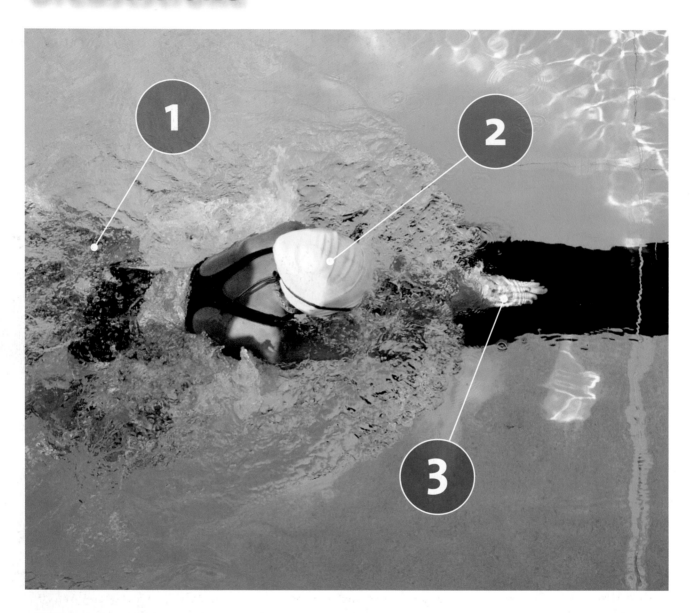

1 Your arms and legs must work at the same time to ensure maximum power, smoothness and balance.

2 Part of your head must be above water for the whole race apart from during the dive phase and the turns.

3 Push the water down and around with your arms to create a turbine effect and maximize forward motion.

Breaststroke can be a difficult stroke to master as it relies on your arms and legs moving simultaneously. If your arms and legs aren't moving simultaneously then the stroke may be illegal and you will be disqualified from the race. Breaststroke also requires the correct timing of your arms and legs to make the stroke efficient. The rules of breaststroke state that except for the underwater arm pull and the leg kick of the start and turn, your head must break the surface of the water during every stroke. Your arms and legs must also be symmetrical.

Body position

Your body position is important in breaststroke: your body should lie flat in the water as you stretch forwards on the recovery of the stroke. Your body's position will change during the stroke as you take a breath and you will need to lift your body up to allow your head to come up to breathe properly.

As your head lifts you should keep your eyes looking down and forwards rather than straight ahead. This helps to stop your body coming up too high, which can lead to your legs and hips dropping too low and creating a lot of resistance in the water. As your head starts to return to the water your arms must stretch forwards so that your body can

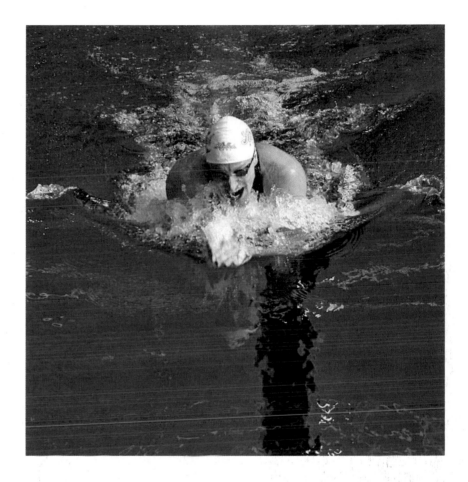

return into the horizontal streamlined position.

Leg kick

The leg recovery phase is when your legs are moved from the streamlined position where they are straight with your toes pointed, to the bent position just before they kick back into the catch phase

During the recovery phase move your legs towards the back of

your thighs and bring your feet up towards your backside while trying to keep your knees at about the width of your hips. It is important that your legs come up towards your backside rather than under your body as that will cause resistance in the water and will slow the stroke down.

As the legs are at the top of the recovery phase your feet should move into the dorsi-flexed position, which is when the feet turn out. Your feet should be positioned slightly wider than your knees to make sure they get strong propulsion. Your legs need to then kick back, around, and then whip in so that they finish in a streamlined position ready to start the next kick.

It is vital for your feet not to break the surface of the water at any time. This will be construed as a 'flutter kick', which is illegal in breaststroke and will lead to instant disqualification.

Arms
Your arms should start in a stream-lined position with the palms of the hands facing outwards so that they are ready to press on the water and start the catch. Your arms should stay straight and start to press outwards until they are just wider than your shoulders. Your hands should then start to turn downwards and inwards as they start to catch the water.

Your elbows must stay high as your hands press down and start to sweep backwards to ensure your forearms are also pressing on the water. Your hands then turn inwards to face each other just below your chest as the propulsion phase finishes and you prepare for the recovery.

There is a slight pause between the propulsion phase and the recovery. As soon as your hands are underneath your chest they should be pushed forwards just below the surface and back into the streamlined position where you can then hold a short glide.

Breathing
Breathing can occur near the start of the pull. As your arms start to press out, your head will start to raise and this is where you can breathe. Your head will go back down just as your arms are

starting to push forwards so that your head is in position as you move back into the streamlined position. Some part of your head must remain above water at all times apart from just after diving.

Timing
Your whole body should be fully stretched at the start of the stroke with your arms starting to pull before your legs start to move. As your arms start the propulsion phase your legs should start to move up towards your backside and as you start to bring back your arms into the recovery phase your legs should be propelling backwards into the propulsion phase. You should then finish back in a streamlined position.

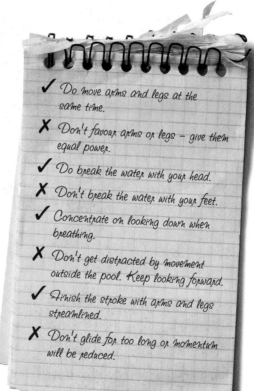

✓ Do move arms and legs at the same time.

✗ Don't favour arms or legs – give them equal power.

✓ Do break the water with your head.

✗ Don't break the water with your feet.

✓ Concentrate on looking down when breathing.

✗ Don't get distracted by movement outside the pool. Keep looking forward.

✓ Finish the stroke with arms and legs streamlined.

✗ Don't glide for too long or momentum will be reduced.

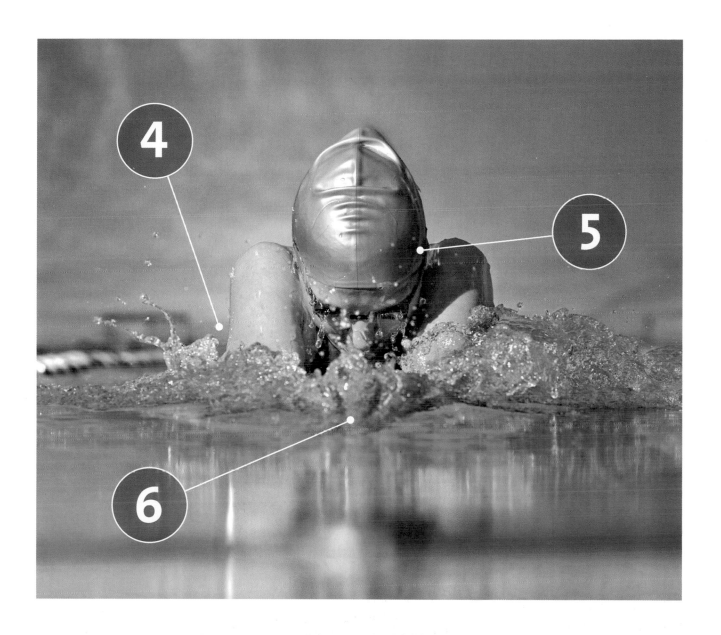

4 Your heels must be kept underwater at all times or you will face disqualification.

5 Look towards the bottom of the pool when breathing out to retain balance.

6 Your arms and legs must finish the stroke fully stretched to ensure you get the furthest glide distance.

Butterfly

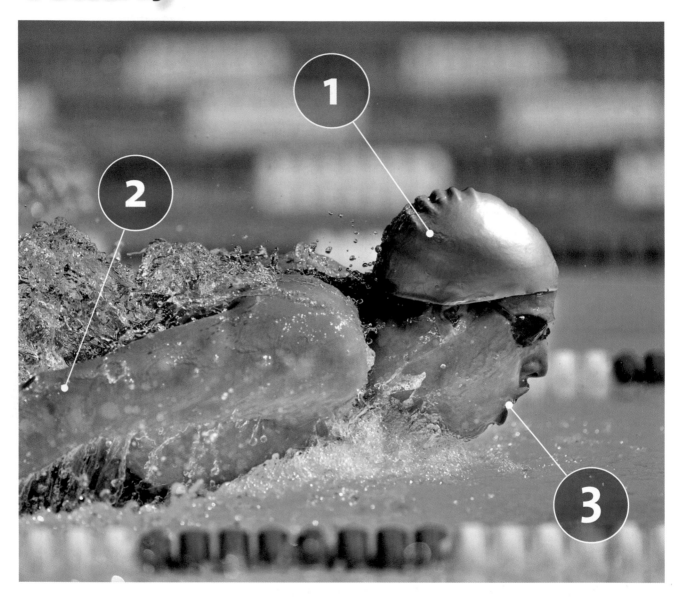

1 Ensure your head is kept low when breathing to give you a smooth stroke.

2 Your elbows must come out of the water ahead of your hands so you pull water with your whole arm strength.

3 Breathe once every other stroke to increase efficiency and maintain oxygen levels.

Butterfly is seen as the toughest of all the four strokes as it is physically the most demanding on your body. It also requires correct timing otherwise it can be even more exhausting. Butterfly can be used to help improve your overall strength in the pool due to its physical demands; many swimmers will swim butterfly for this specific reason even if they are freestyle, backstroke or breaststroke swimmers predominantly.

Body position

You should be horizontal in the water while your hips should stay near the surface. It may look as if professional swimmers are flexing their entire body during the butterfly stroke but in fact they are only bending from the waist.

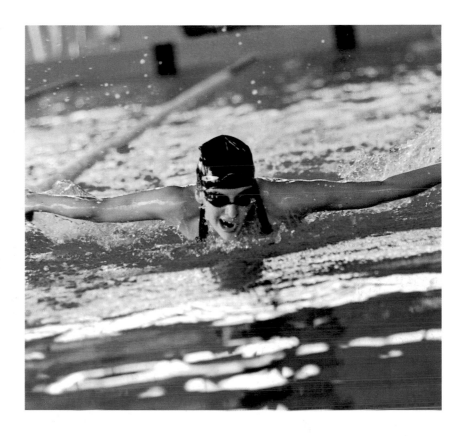

Your head should stay in a central position with your eyes looking down and slightly forwards. You need to try and stay horizontal as the stroke is performed so as to not create too much resistance.

If your legs sink due to a weak leg kick and your head rises too high when breathing, your position in the water will become more vertical, putting more pressure on your arms and reducing efficiency because you are exposing more of your body surface to the water.

Leg kick

The butterfly leg kick is a simultaneous vertical leg kick, known as a 'flutter kick', which requires your feet to move upwards and downwards at the same time. The key to a successful butterfly leg kick is allowing the kick to come from your hips and not purely from the knees, which is a common mistake.

During the 'up' phase of the kick your knees should be slightly flexed to allow your feet to move upwards towards the surface of the water

until your toes break the surface. At this point your feet need to be fully extended from the ankle all the way to the toes. At this stage your hips should be moving slightly downwards to stop your knees having to flex too much.

As your legs start the down phase of the kick your legs and feet should quickly push down on the water, which will make the hips push up towards the surface of the water creating the undulating body motion. Your legs should be straight at this point as they start to move back into the upwards kick.

Arms

Your hands' entry is the start of the stroke's catch, which leads into the propulsion phase of the arm stroke. Your hands need to enter with the palms facing diagonally downwards, with your arms stretched in front at about shoulder width. As your hands enter the water they should press outwards and downwards in a sculling motion before starting to press backwards.

Your elbows should be kept high in the water as this first phase of the arm stroke occurs. As your arms start to press backwards they should travel in the direction of your stomach with your hands almost meeting underneath before sweeping back out, with your hands exiting the water past the hips. It is vital for a good butterfly stroke that you keep your elbows high during the pull phase to ensure you have a powerful stroke.

Your hands should always be below your elbows as the arms are pulling through the water. Your elbows should be the first part of your arms to exit the water, quickly followed by your hands. Your arms are then relaxed as they recover forward together with your thumbs pointing down towards the bottom of the pool back to where the hands enter the water again.

Breathing

Breathing occurs during the start of the pull phase of the stroke with your head being raised while trying to keep your chin low to the water. Your head should then be returned back into position as soon as you have taken a breath and before your hands enter the water.

If your head is raised too high when breathing it will disrupt

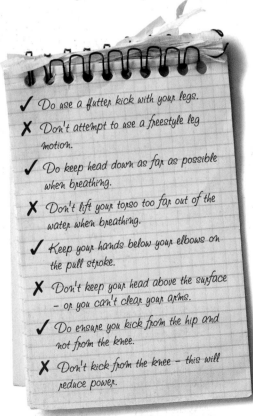

- ✓ Do use a flutter kick with your legs.
- ✗ Don't attempt to use a freestyle leg motion.
- ✓ Do keep head down as far as possible when breathing.
- ✗ Don't lift your torso too far out of the water when breathing.
- ✓ Keep your hands below your elbows on the pull stroke.
- ✗ Don't keep your head above the surface – or you can't clear your arms.
- ✓ Do ensure you kick from the hip and not from the knee.
- ✗ Don't kick from the knee – this will reduce power.

the rhythm of the stroke. The key is to keep yourself low to the water and keep the whole breathing cycle smooth so as to not interrupt the stroke. You should take one breath for every two strokes – if you leave it longer your body will become oxygen deprived because butterfly is such a demanding discipline.

Timing

Your legs should kick twice during each arm cycle, with the first occurring right at the start of the stroke, which is just after your hands enter the water and start the catch phase. The second kick occurs as your arms are preparing to leave the water. If your head is out of the water during the whole recovery phase it makes it more difficult to get the arms over the water. This is the part of the stroke some people struggle with.

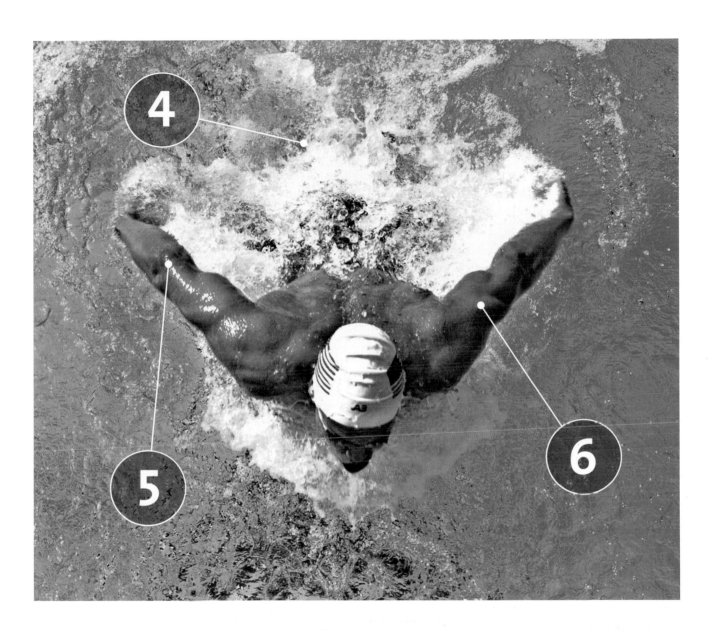

4 Both your legs must kick at the same time – not as in a freestyle leg kick, which is outlawed in butterfly.

5 Keep your elbows raised during the pull stroke to give you extra power.

6 Maintain a rhythm of one arm cycle to two leg cycles.

Freestyle

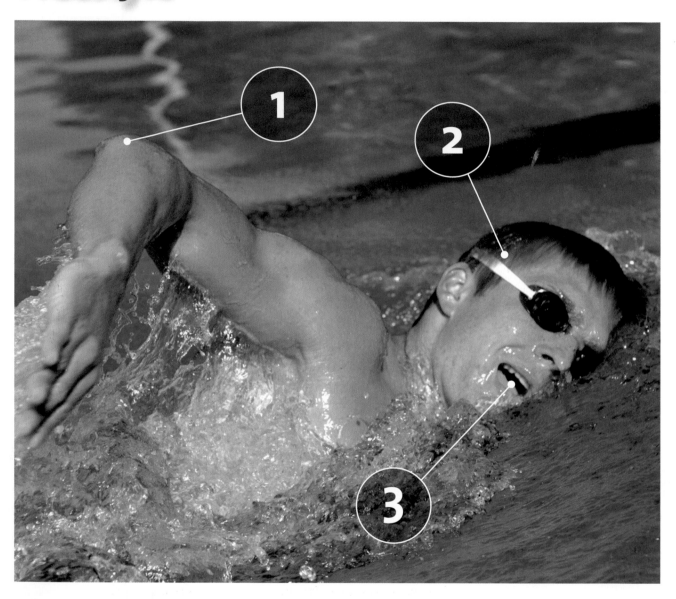

1 Get your elbows out of the water first – this lets you stretch further for maximum pull.

2 Put in a complete 90-degree head turn for each breath so you don't swallow water.

3 Breathing every three strokes is the best to get the most out of race (unless you are a sprinter).

Body position

Head: your head should be positioned with your eyes looking at approximately 45 degrees to the water's surface with the water hitting the crown of your head. It is important your head remains still between breathing to help maintain your body's streamlined position.

Head position during breathing: your head should turn 90 degrees when you are breathing. It is important to make sure your head turns as little as possible so that you minimize the disturbance to your body's streamlined position. Your head rotation will be assisted by your upper body's rotation; timing is key in ensuring your head turns as your shoulders rotate.

Hips and upper body: your shoulders should rotate to help keep the stroke long and to ensure that your body is streamlined at all times. As your hand enters the water one shoulder will drop while your other shoulder will rotate in the opposite direction.

Your shoulders should rotate to around 45 degrees to the surface of the water, which will reduce the surface area of your body as it travels through the water. Your hips should follow through the rotation of your shoulders.

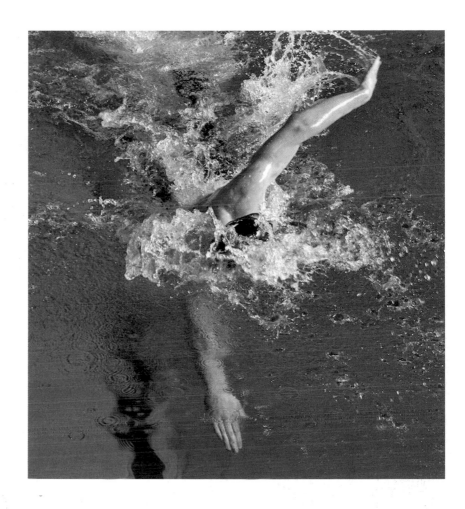

Leg kick

The freestyle leg kick is important because it helps you to maintain your body's position in the water as well as aiding your forward propulsion. A strong leg kick will help you to maintain your body's position at the surface of the water.

A six-beat kick is commonly used by swimmers, which means six kicks to every two arm strokes or one complete arm cycle. Your legs should be kept long with minimal knee flexion, with the kick coming from your hip and your ankles loose with toes pointed.

Hand entry

Your hand should be rotated to a 45-degree angle as it enters the water with your finger tips entering before any other part of the hand. By entering the water with your hands at this angle they will be in the position to start the out sweep at the start of the pull. Your hand should enter as far from your head as possible to help ensure you have a long stroke.

Arms

Once your hand has entered the water, try to maintain a high elbow during the pull phase of the stroke. Your arms should start sweeping in an outward and downward direction. Then pull inwards and upwards just before the stroke pushes backwards, with your fingers exiting past the hip.

As your arm exits the water your elbow should be kept high and your hand close to your body as your other arm starts the pull phase. As your arm recovers over the water your elbow should be kept high with your fingers close to the water's surface as your arm stretches out over the water for a long hand entry.

Breathing

Swimmers have used different breathing patterns for freestyle swimming over the years, such as every two, three or four strokes and also combinations such as 2-2-3 and 4-4-2.

The most common breathing pattern is every three strokes. This is known as bilateral breathing, which ensures regular oxygen intake without breaking your body's streamlined position too often to breathe. Breathing every two strokes will mean the stroke's streamlined position is broken more frequently, whereas when breathing every four or five strokes the stroke is kept streamlined for more of the swim but you will oxygenate less frequently.

Different breathing patterns have their use in different freestyle events. For example, sprinters will breathe fewer times – in a 50-metre race top swimmers will breathe once at the most – as they are trying to maintain the streamlined position and don't require as much oxygen as others. In middle-distance races, swimmers breathe every five or six strokes.

Distance swimming will require a more frequent oxygen supply so breathing bilaterally every three strokes is often used in longer events with the added bonus that you can keep an eye on your opponents' progress as you come up to breathe.

✓ Breathe every two or more strokes.

✗ Don't try to breathe on every stroke – it wastes momentum.

✓ Breathe to the side and fully turn your head to maximize oxygen intake.

✗ Don't try to get your head fully out of the water when breathing.

✓ Do let your fingertips enter the water first on the pull stroke.

✗ Don't let your hands hit the water close to your head.

✓ Stretch your arms as fully as possible on the pull stroke.

✗ Don't kick from the knee – kick from the hip.

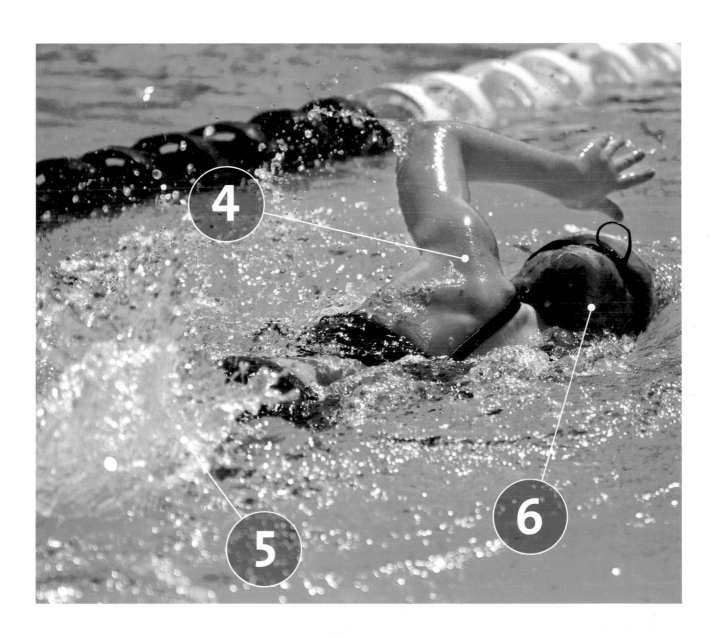

4 Keep the stroke long and efficient by rotating your shoulders and your hips will follow.

5 Use a six-beat freestyle kick – that is six kicks for one complete arm cycle.

6 Keep your head at 45 degrees to the surface to reduce drag and to maintain momentum.

Starts – backstroke

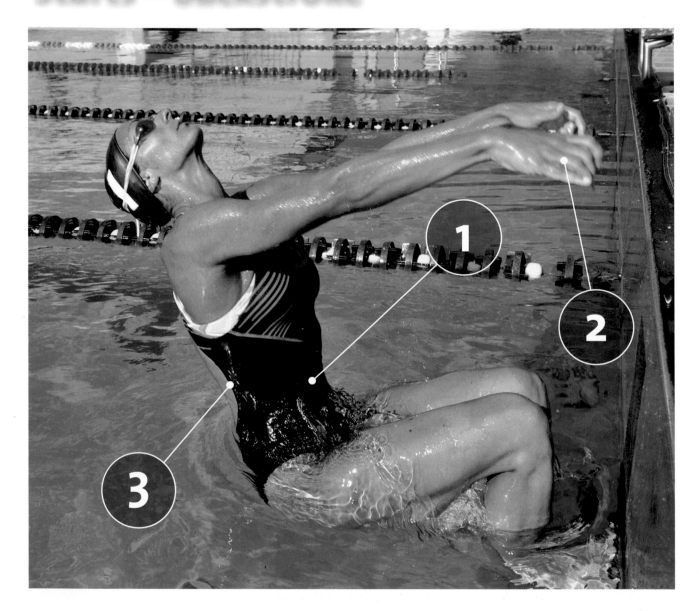

1 You should be like a coiled spring as you cling to the wall to ensure maximum height out of the water at the start.

2 Push your hands out as far as possible when pushing off to lengthen your stroke.

3 Go over the water, not through it, when you push off. You are quicker through air than through water.

For the backstroke start you will be starting in the water with both your feet positioned on the wall while you are holding the bar that is on the block. You should then pull yourself into the wall to prepare to give yourself the maximum power for the takeoff. As with the start off the blocks it only takes one false start and you will be out of the competition. Your feet should be positioned on the wall at about shoulder width apart or just slightly less than this. You can either start with both feet level or in a slight track stance with one foot higher than the other.

Stages of the backstroke start

1. The referee blows the whistle to indicate you can enter the water. Most top competitors will dive conventionally into the pool, swim as far as the flags and return to the wall using backstroke to count how many strokes it is back to the wall. This will help them with their finish and turns in the actual race. They then get themselves into the start position.

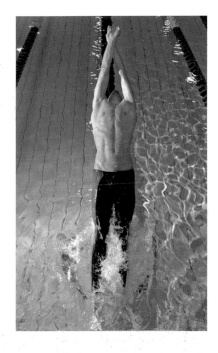

2. The starter will then say "Take your marks". At this point you should pull yourself towards the block with your arms (with your feet still positioned on the wall) using the balls of your feet as the main contact to aid a springy start.

3. As soon as the starting signal goes, throw your arms backwards into a streamlined position and use your legs to push off the wall. Arch your back as you push backwards to make sure you travel over the water rather than through it.

4. You should now be in a stream-lined position under the water, with one hand on top of the other above your head, and you should be flutter kicking. As you approach the surface you should start backstroke kicking, while maintaining your hands in this streamlined position, until they break the water. As with all other strokes, the 15-metre rule applies, at which point you must be up and swimming backstroke.

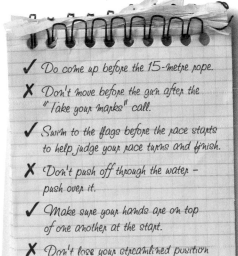

✓ Do come up before the 15-metre rope.

✗ Don't move before the gun after the "Take your marks" call.

✓ Swim to the flags before the race starts to help judge your pace turns and finish.

✗ Don't push off through the water – push over it.

✓ Make sure your hands are on top of one another at the start.

✗ Don't lose your streamlined position until you break the surface.

Starts – blocks

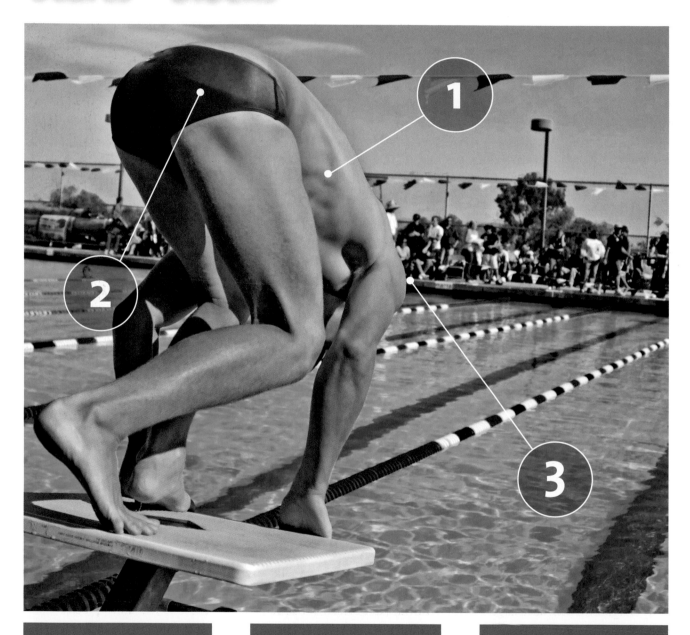

1 When you hear the order "Take your marks", take your position and don't move again until you hear the gun.

2 Keep your backside as the highest point of your body on the block with your legs slightly bent.

3 Keep your head down – if you lose your goggles on the dive you will have difficulty seeing where you are going throughout the race.

You can't win a race with your dive, but you can lose it with a poor one. The race is the culmination of all that time in the training pool, so why waste all of that hard training with a slow start?

The best starters can steal a march on their opponents, a potentially demoralizing blow for the sluggish, but if you are too quick out of the blocks you will be disqualified. Once the referee has blown his whistle to signal you onto the blocks you will have about 10 seconds before the action starts.

During this time you need to look down your lane at the spot where you will hit the water, like a golfer sizing up his opening drive at the Open Championship, or a tennis player eyeing up a serve at Wimbledon. Briefly run through your race strategy and training drills and, to dispel pre-race nerves, imagine yourself on the podium a few minutes later. Some top competitors use the moments before they race to indulge in mind games with the other swimmers to try and gain a crucial advantage on the blocks. Then it is "Take your marks, go..." Once you hit the water you must be above the surface by the 15-metre rope or you will be disqualified and all your hard work will be undone.

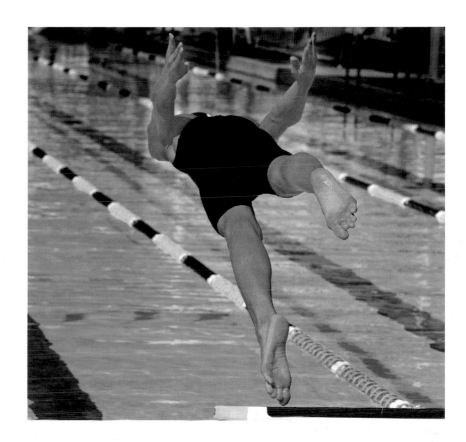

The Dive

There are two main types of dive: the grab start and the track start. Both have advantages and disadvantages but the most important thing to remember is you only get one chance. If you false start once you are immediately disqualified – with no exceptions. In the 2008 Beijing Olympics, Australia's Libby Trickett was the beneficiary of hometown favourite Pang Jiaying's disqualification in the semi-finals of the 100-metre freestyle due to a false start. Trickett went on to win the silver medal in a final she may not even have been in if Jiaying had not infringed the rules.

Referees can hold competitors on the blocks after the "Take your marks" order for as long as they like. They mix it up from race to race so you cannot predict the gun and gain an advantage. Some coaches try to analyze each referee's habits to help their swimmers jump the gun but they are treading a fine line with the penalty of instant disqualification awaiting the competitor if they get it slightly wrong.

The grab start is where you have both feet at the front of the block with your toes curled over the edge. Your feet should be positioned at about shoulder width apart with your hands stretched down in a streamlined position grabbing the block in between your feet. Your head should be down, with your backside at the highest point and your legs slightly bent. The grab start is seen as a powerful start because the energy is concentrated into a smaller area than with the track start.

For the track start you take a stance on the block similar to that adopted by a middle-distance runner, with one foot forward in line with one shoulder. The toes of your front foot should be curled over the edge of the block. Your other foot is in line with your other shoulder but moved to the back of the block.

Your head should be down and your toes should be holding onto the front of the block, which they can pull against to get tension in the muscles. The track start is sometimes seen as less powerful but is a good start to get a fast reaction off the block. It can reduce your chances of a false start because you are more balanced than with the grab start.

Stages of the dive

1. The referee will blow the whistle, which indicates you can get up on the blocks.
2. You then get your feet into position ready for the referee's start order.
3. The referee will then say, "Take your marks", which is when you get into your start position. Once you have set your position you are not allowed to move until the starting signal.
4. The referee will initiate the starting signal, then you are allowed to leave the block which you should do in a streamlined position, entering the water fingers first.
5. It is important to keep your head down and not look forwards as you enter the water to ensure your goggles don't slip.

Freestyle, breaststroke and butterfly all have unique techniques once the you hit the water – but you must remember the 15-metre rule and the technique for each stroke because in competition there will be up to eight officials policing the pool.

In freestyle you should flutter kick until you are about to break the surface. Then switch to a freestyle leg kick and start swimming. In breaststroke you can make a maximum of one arm pull and one leg kick underwater, then break the water as you start the second stroke.

In butterfly, similar to freestyle, swimmers flutter kick to the surface and start swimming.

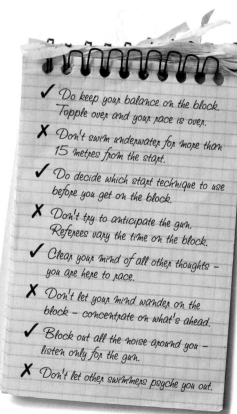

✔ Do keep your balance on the block. Topple over and your race is over.

✘ Don't swim underwater for more than 15 metres from the start.

✔ Do decide which start technique to use before you get on the block.

✘ Don't try to anticipate the gun. Referees vary the time on the block.

✔ Clear your mind of all other thoughts – you are here to race.

✘ Don't let your mind wander on the block – concentrate on what's ahead.

✔ Block out all the noise around you – listen only for the gun.

✘ Don't let other swimmers psyche you out.

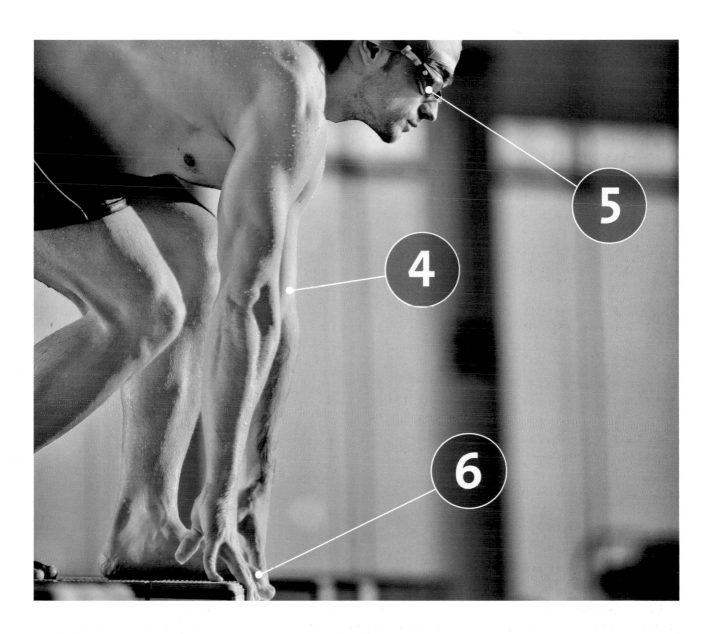

4 A false start means disqualification so maintain your balance on the block.

5 Remember to focus on the race – maintain your concentration and look ahead.

6 Grab the block with your toes as it gets your muscles ready for action.

Turns – backstroke

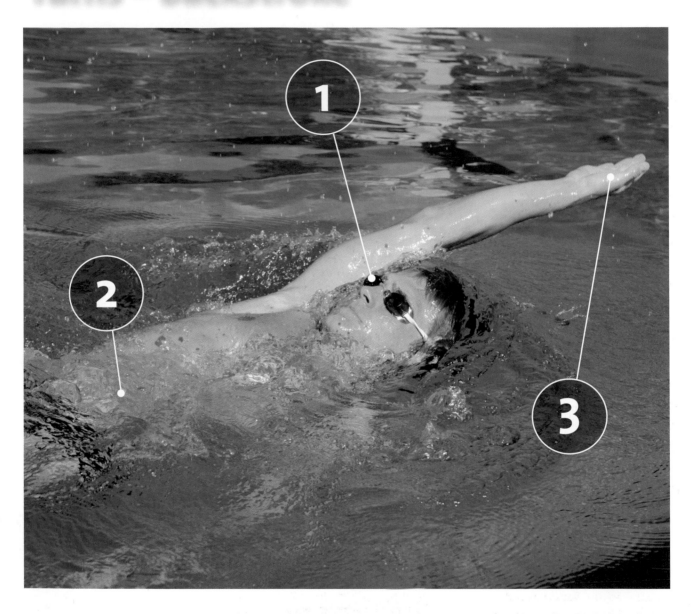

1 Always count the distance between the flags and the wall ahead of racing.

2 Try to turn onto your stomach on a full stroke as the arm guides the turn.

3 Turn as close to the wall as possible to maximize the distance of your push off.

At first sight this is probably the hardest turn of the lot to execute because you are going backwards as you approach the wall and cannot see it. However, there are ways around this. Conveniently for all backstrokers there are flags placed above that give a guide as to how far it is to the wall. The basic principle is to stay as tight to the wall as possible to increase the spring in your push off.

Approach

The backstroke turn is very similar to the freestyle turn, apart from the obvious point that your approach is on your back and you need to turn onto your front before turning.

Many swimmers are apprehensive at the thought of swimming into a wall 'blind', but with a bit of preparation, by measuring the distance between the flags and the wall, you can easily avoid a potentially nerve-racking situation. The more times you do this successfully the more your confidence will grow.

As you reach the flags you need to know how many strokes to take from the flags to the wall. You then count these strokes out as you are swimming and then, one stroke before you reach the wall, you should flip onto your front for the turn.

Rotation

Once you have turned onto your front your arm needs to come over to start the rotation. Whether you turn left or right depends on which arm is leading the stroke into the wall. Your head should start to tuck in as your legs flip over the top and your feet should be placed on the wall ready to push off for the next length. As on the freestyle turn it is important to keep the whole rotation smooth and to tuck in as tight as you can to make the changeover at the end of the pool as fast as possible.

Leaving the wall

Now that your feet are placed on the wall you can push off into a tight streamlined position, with your hands outstretched and placed one on top of the other, as they should have been when you were starting the race. From this position you should flutter kick underwater until you are about to break the surface, which is when you should switch to the backstroke kick and start swimming full stroke as the race continues.

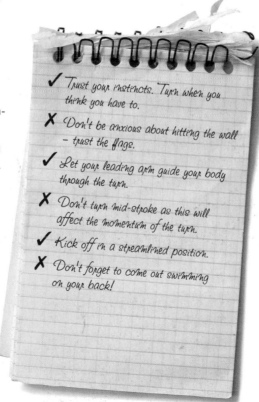

✓ Trust your instincts. Turn when you think you have to.

✗ Don't be anxious about hitting the wall – trust the flags.

✓ Let your leading arm guide your body through the turn.

✗ Don't turn mid-stroke as this will affect the momentum of the turn.

✓ Kick off in a streamlined position.

✗ Don't forget to come out swimming on your back!

Turns – freestyle

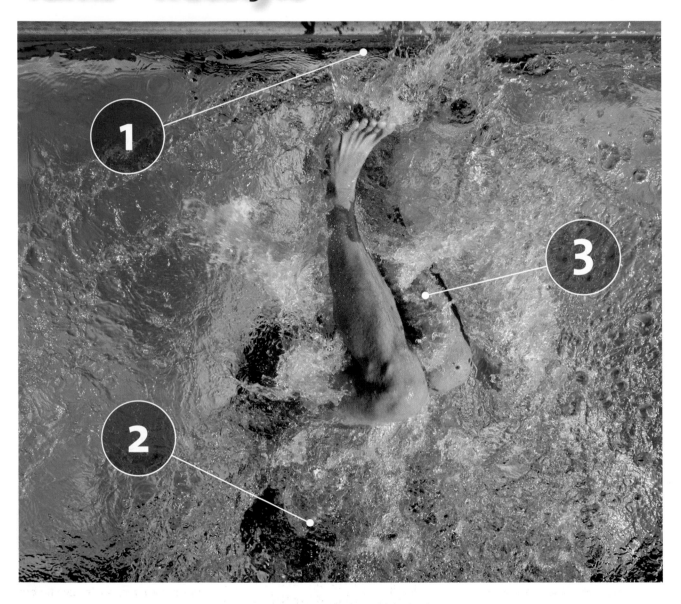

1 Swim as close to the wall as possible as this gives you the best chance of a more powerful push off.

2 Make sure both arms are under the water so they can initiate the head turn and your legs will follow.

3 As you turn keep your legs tucked in to reduce water resistance, which give you a quicker rotation.

Many novices are fearful of performing a tumble turn for the first time. The thought of somersaulting upside down underwater is alien to natural land dwellers, but with practice it can make the difference between winning and losing a race at any level. In a 200-metre race you turn three times and every poor turn can mean seconds onto your time. Professional swimmers know the importance of the turn. They spend countless hours perfecting their technique in the training pool because at the top level even a hundredth of a second can be the difference between the gold medal and fourth place.

Timing is crucial. If your turn is too long you will have to return and touch the wall before setting off on the next length or face disqualification. If your turn is too short your legs will be over the side of the pool and the whole rhythm of your race disrupted. The very best turners can curl themselves up into a tight ball as they turn giving themselves spring and the maximum power off the wall and a crucial advantage over their opponents.

Approach

The first part of the turn is the approach where you near the wall. With practice you will subconsciously know when to begin your turn – although exactly where you will start to initiate the action depends on your height and flexibility. Shorter swimmers can turn closer to the wall as can the most flexible. It is important you approach the wall at a good speed so you can turn quickly. The last stroke becomes the tumble turn as you start to drop your head and tuck it into your chest as you take your last stroke leading into the turn.

✓ Do turn on completion of a full stroke – it makes life easier.

✗ Don't turn too far away from the wall and risk disqualification.

✓ Do keep up your speed going into the wall before turning.

✗ Don't let your arms come out of the water during the turn.

✓ Do keep as streamlined a position as possible as you leave the wall.

✗ Don't be scared – just turn...

The Rotation

As you take your last stroke and are starting to tuck your head in, take a final breath if you need it before the turn. Keep both arms under the water and start to rotate head first with your legs flipping over the top of your head. You should try to keep your legs tucked in tight as you turn to help speed up the rotation. Then position your feet on the wall ready for the push off. At this point you should be as tight to the wall as possible to ensure a powerful push off from the wall.

Leaving the wall

With your feet now positioned on the wall you need to get your arms into a streamlined position before the push off. When you are as close to the wall as you can get push off as explosively as possible and go into a streamlined position underwater. From there, flutter kick underwater, remembering the 15-metre rule about swimming beneath the surface also applies to turns, before reaching the surface. Just below the surface you should switch to a freestyle leg kick before getting into the full swimming stroke and on with the business of racing.

Turns – breaststroke & butterfly

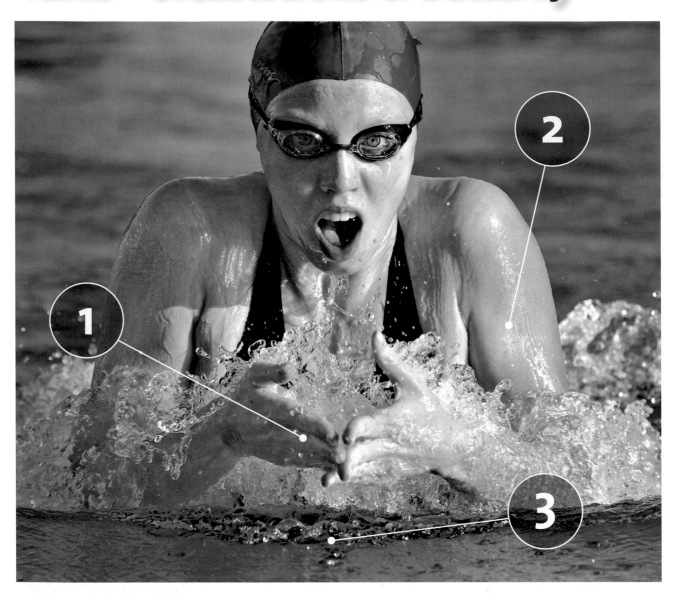

1 Touch the wall with two hands at the same time or it is not a legal turn.

2 Use your leading arm to guide you through the turn and let your body follow.

3 Swim into the wall as fast as possible – this generates momentum through the turn and gives you more power out of it.

The breaststroke and butterfly

turns are very similar in that they both require finishing on a full stroke and touching the wall with two hands. The rule is that you must touch the wall with two hands at the same time or be disqualified. The only difference between the two turns is the last stroke into the wall and what happens when you leave the wall.

Approach

You need to approach the wall swimming a full stroke and (for butterfly) keeping your head down

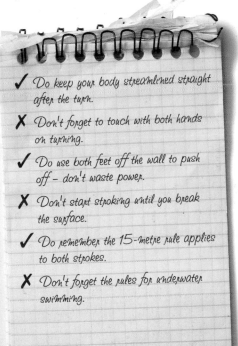

✓ Do keep your body streamlined straight after the turn.

✗ Don't forget to touch with both hands on turning.

✓ Do use both feet off the wall to push off – don't waste power.

✗ Don't start stroking until you break the surface.

✓ Do remember the 15-metre rule applies to both strokes.

✗ Don't forget the rules for underwater swimming.

on the last couple of strokes into the wall so as to not disturb your stroke rhythm. Again, you should be looking to swim into the wall as fast as possible. It is important you hit the wall with both hands at speed with your hands positioned at about shoulder width apart so that the judge can clearly see both hands touch the wall. The speed that you swim into the wall with will be transferred into the speed of the turn, hence the importance of not slowing down into the wall.

Rotation

Once you have touched the wall you should keep your eyes fixed on your hands as you bring your legs underneath from behind your body. As your feet approach the wall your leading arm should pull away from the wall and point in the direction of where you intend to push off, while you are still keeping your eyes fixed on the wall. As soon as your feet plant on the wall at about shoulder width or slightly less you are ready to leave the wall.

Breaststroke leaving the wall

You should leave the wall in a streamlined position with your eyes looking down. You should be horizontal as you leave the wall, holding the streamlined pose as you first leave the wall and hold

for approximately three seconds before then starting the single arm pull that is permitted underwater on starts and turns on breaststroke. Your arms should sweep out then around, then back, and finish by your hips, a position you should hold momentarily.

As your arms start to recover under your body you should return to a streamlined position while your legs initiate the first leg kick, which is also allowed off the start and turns. You must then wait to break the surface before starting to swim full stroke otherwise you will be disqualified. It is important to remember that you are only allowed one arm pull and one leg kick underwater at the start and turns.

Butterfly leaving the wall

You should leave the wall in a streamlined position with your body slightly on its side at approximately a 45-degree angle. As you start the flutter kick you should rotate onto your front facing the bottom of the pool and kick until you are at the surface ready to swim. You should then break out into full stroke and keep your head down for the first two or three full strokes.

Finishes – backstroke

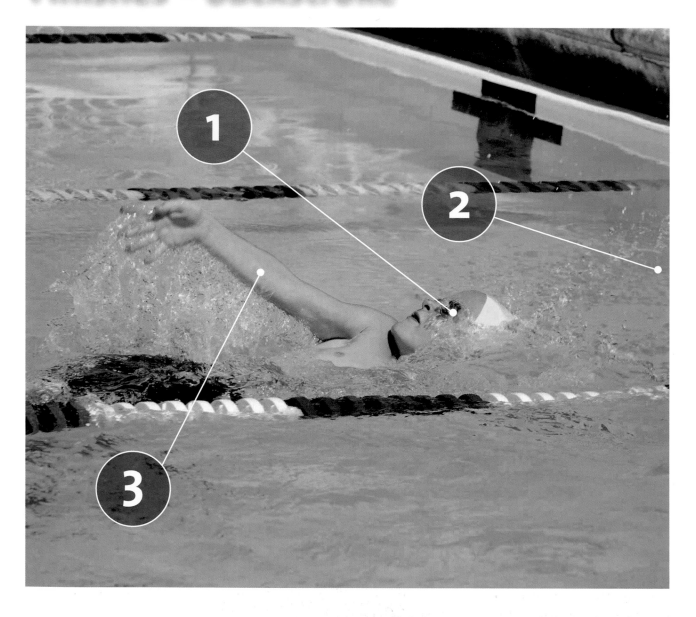

1 Do count the flags before you touch the wall and keep swimming hard until you reach it.

2 Don't search for the wall – it will arrive soon enough.

3 Make sure you finish your race on a full stroke to shave vital fractions off your time.

Finishes

Finishing a race is not as simple as it sounds and it is certainly not just a matter of touching the wall. Many tight races have been lost by swimmers getting just short of the wall at the end of a stroke, then having to glide in to touch for glory and therefore losing momentum and the race in the process.

The perfect finish to a race comes when you can touch the wall at the precise moment your full stroke finishes. Top-level performers will know that a slightly short stroke, as they near the wall, followed by a full one, will give them the optimum finishing position and they will work hard on this technique for extra finishing power.

As you approach the last stroke, stretch yourself as far as you possibly can and rotate your body onto its side. This puts you in a more streamlined position thus saving valuable milliseconds. It is things like this which can make all the difference. You should use everything you can to your advantage in a race, even small tips like this!

Backstroke

As you approach the wall you should not let your stroke rhythm slow down, and whatever happens, do not start looking around for the finish – that's what the flags are for and that's what you need to trust. You should stretch back on the last stroke in a strong positive manner so you are able to touch the wall as quickly as possible.

Breaststroke and butterfly

In butterfly, as you are approaching the last five metres of the race, you should aim to keep your head down so you do not disturb the rhythm of your strokes and in order to keep your speed as high as possible. For both breaststroke and butterfly

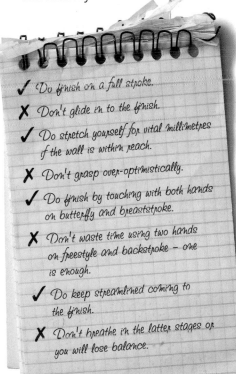

- ✓ Do finish on a full stroke.
- ✗ Don't glide in to the finish.
- ✓ Do stretch yourself for vital millimetres if the wall is within reach.
- ✗ Don't grasp over-optimistically.
- ✓ Do finish by touching with both hands on butterfly and breaststroke.
- ✗ Don't waste time using two hands on freestyle and backstroke – one is enough.
- ✓ Do keep streamlined coming to the finish.
- ✗ Don't breathe in the latter stages or you will lose balance.

strokes, as you approach the last stroke coming into the wall you should stretch at full length as your hands move through the water while remembering to always keep your head down. You must touch with two hands simultaneously for a legitimate finish in these strokes. Don't ruin a good race with a mistake right at the end by touching with one hand.

Freestyle

Try not breathe in the last five or 10 metres as this disrupts the rhythm of your stroke and slows you down as you head into the business end of the race. A touch with any part of one hand is legal.

Finishes – breaststroke & butterfly

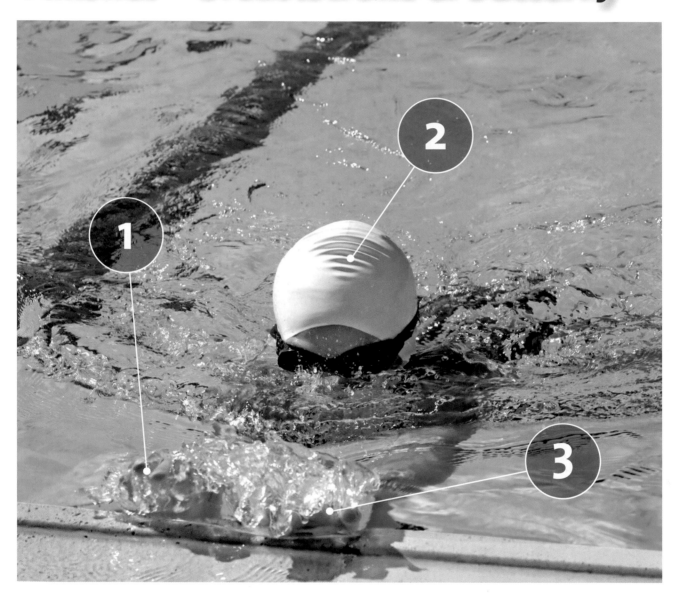

1 You must touch the wall with both hands for the finish to be legal. Timing is the key.

2 Keep your head down as you near the finish otherwise your balance will suffer.

3 Always try to touch on a full stroke – don't glide in and lose your momentum.

Finishes – freestyle

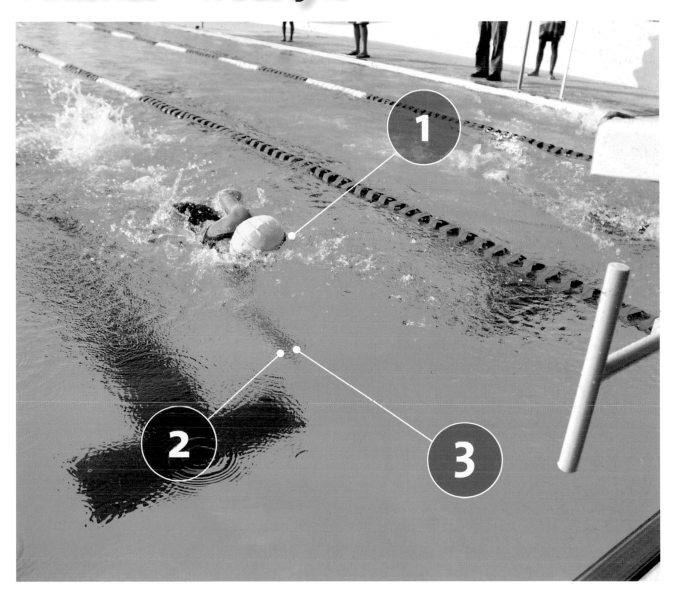

1 Try not to breathe in the closing stages of the race – there is plenty of time for that later.

2 Don't glide for the wall – lunge for it. This can make all the difference.

3 Any part of your hand counts when touching the wall – even your little finger!

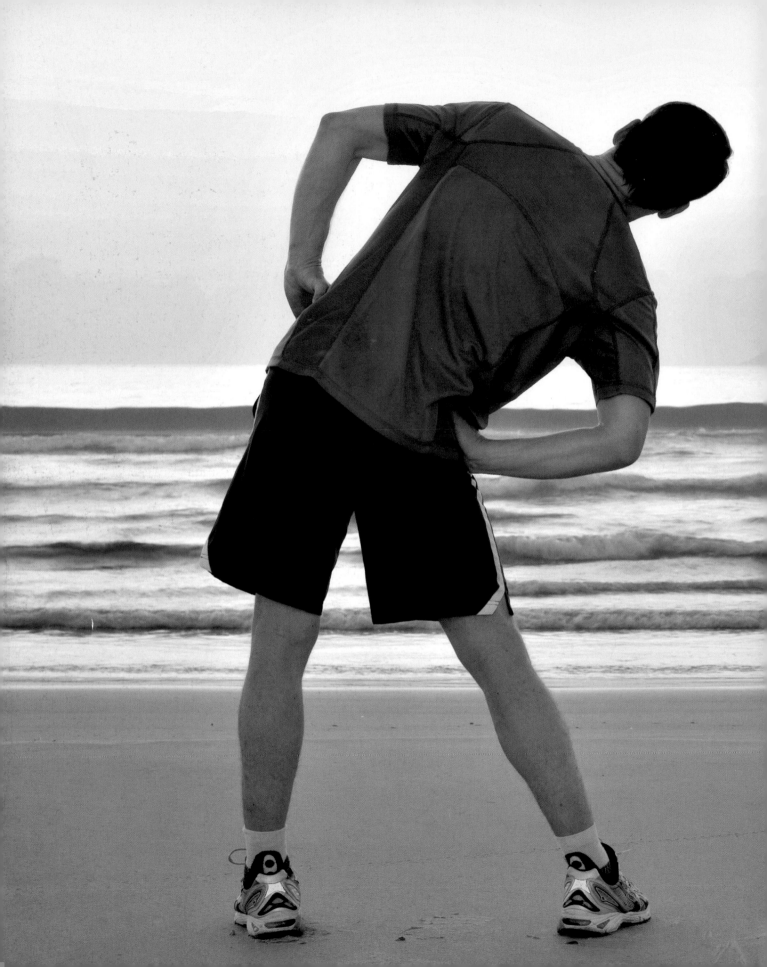

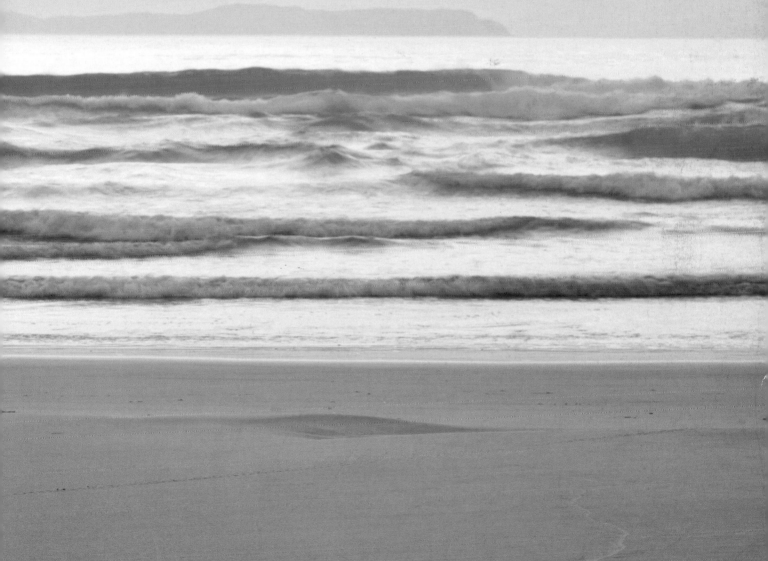

fitness & training

// FASTER // FITTER // MORE MOTIVATED

Training zones

Training zones allow you to work at the correct intensity. When starting a training session it is important to know the reason you are training. What is your goal for this session and what do you want your mind and body to achieve? It is unrealistic to think that you can push your body 100 per cent every time you enter the pool. This is why training programmes start with a light workload and then have gradual increases. Even as the workload increases there will still be some lighter weeks that allow your body to recover.

A lot of your planning will depend on your training history. If you have prepared for an event before you will be more aware of what your body can sustain without suffering adverse affects. If this is the first time you are undertaking a more structured training programme, or if you are training for a new event, you should try to follow the training programme you set out and take care not to get carried away (See Over-training and over-reaching on page 72).

There are also many positive aspects for working at the correct intensities. Improving different areas of training zones will enable you to get faster and stronger for longer periods, both mentally and physically. Working in the correct training zones allows you, even if you are training by yourself with little or no support, to prepare as the professionals do.

A lot of what we set out in this section is based around heart-rate monitors. If you are training without a heart-rate monitor then you will need to use what we call Rate of Perceived Exertion (RPE). Imagine a scale of one to 10. One is little or no effort, while 10 would be your maximum effort. Where a heart-rate percentage is displayed, simply divide the figure by 10 to get the correct figure for yourself (eg 70-80 per cent of maximum heart rate would equate to 7-8 RPE).

Your heart-rate monitor will normally work out correct training intensities automatically for you. The equation below is included for those monitors that don't and also so you have some background information as to what the monitors are doing.

220 - your age - your resting heart rate. Intensity per cent + resting heart rate = target training zone

For example: an athlete who is aged 30 and has a resting heart rate of 70 beats per minute (bpm) training at 70 per cent of his maximum heart rate is calculated as follows:

220 - 30 - 70 = 120
70 per cent of 120 = 84 + 70 = 154 bpm

It is important to remember that you know your body better than your heart-rate monitor so if you are feeling very ill or dizzy and your heart rate is still low you may need to listen to your body, take down the intensity or even stop. You should also be aware that before aiming for your target training zones you should you be fully warmed up and allow time for your heart rate to climb to the training levels.

Endurance work
60-75 per cent of maximum heart rate

This intensity will normally make up the bulk of your work. You may also hear this referred to as the fat-burning zone, base training or train don't strain. With good technique and an injury-free body you should be able to sustain long periods of time in this training zone.

At this lower intensity level your body can cope with large volumes of time training. Your body should not be put under too much strain, allowing you to concentrate on perfecting technique. It is in this

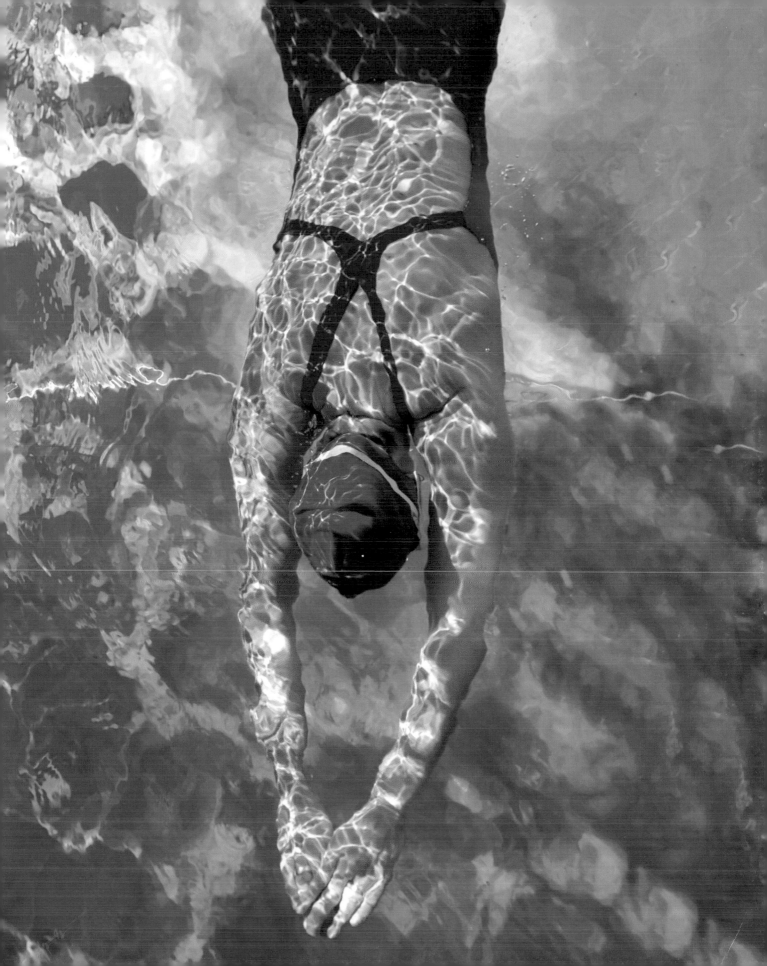

zone that you will be putting in the long hours in the pool and this creates a really good base for your training as well as your body. Physically your body benefits from a stronger heart, the increased ability to take oxygen on-board and using this oxygen more efficiently to help the body perform better. By repeating the correct action of your swimming discipline your muscles will remember what to do and in times of fatigue this can really help to sustain good technique, which will maximize speed and efficiency.

It is also in this training zone that your body will burn high levels of fat. By working at the lower intensity levels the main source of energy your body uses will be fat. Because you can sustain this lower level for longer periods of time and your main fuel is body fat, this equates to a lot of body-fat burning.

This is good news for most people and it can be very rewarding to see your body-fat percentage lower, as well as making you a better performer. After a sustained period of training sessions you will also notice that you can swim further while keeping your heart rate in the same training zone. For some people this happens remarkably fast and it can be really motivating to see the rewards so quickly.

Anaerobic/lactate thresholds
80-90 per cent of maximum heart rate

The above percentages really are just a guideline. The only way to truly establish your exact lactate thresholds is to be tested in a lab. Obviously many of us do not have this option as it can be expensive and requires taking blood.

Your next best option is to do a time trial of your own. Set a distance that is challenging to complete over a 30-minute period and then take your average heart rate over this period. If you feel halfway through the swim that you cannot continue due to muscle fatigue, or your muscles are 'burning', stop and see what your heart rate is as this can be a good indicator as to your lactate threshold.

What's happening and why does it matter? Without becoming too complicated, when training at these levels of intensity, the main source of energy used is glycogen (which is stored in the muscles). A by-product of this is the release of lactate acid. Once this lactate acid accumulates to a certain level your performance will become greatly reduced. So by training at the correct levels it is possible to increase your thresholds and your body can then deal with

the release of the lactate acid more efficiently.

This type of training can greatly enhance your performance. Although it will be less in volume to the endurance work, training around these thresholds can give you the ability to cover longer distances at a faster pace with a lower heart rate. This lower heart rate means that you will produce less lactate acid and can continue with less muscle fatigue. You will be greatly surprised at the gains your body can make in these training levels.

Red-line zone
90-100 per cent of maximum heart rate

This zone is rarely used for endurance athletes. It is mainly used for speed and interval training and can only be sustained for short periods, even if you are very fit. Points to note are that the heart rate can be increased by other factors and may cause you to adjust your training zones accordingly. Dehydration, heat and altitude can all cause the heart rate to increase anywhere between seven to 10 per cent.

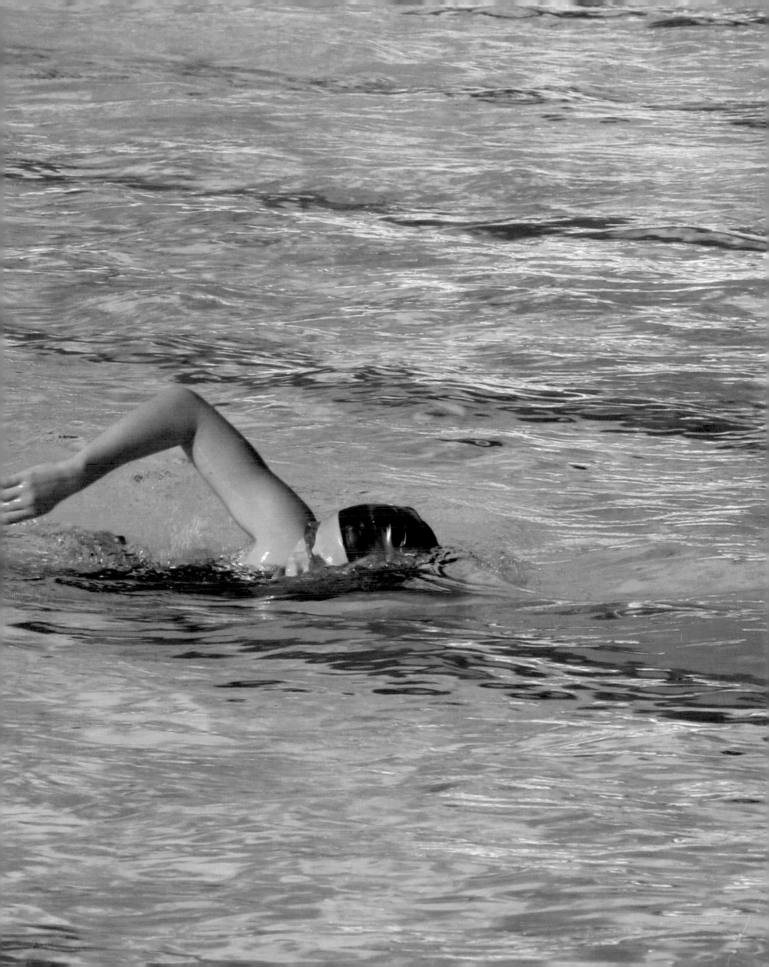

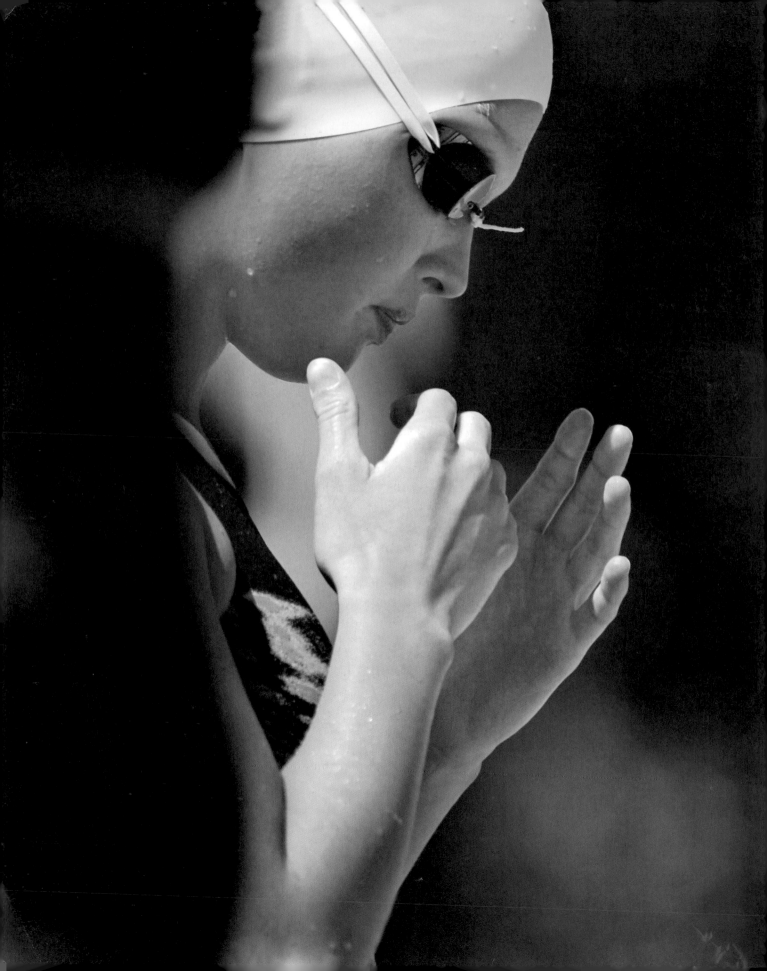

Mental fitness and motivation

It is very common when starting a new project like training for a swimming event for the first time to be full of enthusiasm as you prepare your programmes and throw yourself into the early training sessions. This enthusiasm can quickly wane, leaving you flat and demotivated.

What precautions can you take to help prevent this? Number one: set yourself realistic targets. Your target may just be to complete an event, or you may set yourself a certain time to finish your distance. Whatever your target is, it should be challenging but it must also be achievable.

You will also need to be flexible in your target setting. You may have unforeseen circumstances like an injury, which will make it difficult to train properly for a period of time. The best thing to do is review your challenges and restructure. You may be still on course for your targets, but if you feel you can no longer achieve them you will need to readjust.

When setting your programme make certain you are realistic about the amount of time and energy you can spend training. If you set a schedule with an unrealistic eight training sessions a week, you will inevitably miss some sessions. This is incredibly demotivating, will cause you to stutter in your training and eventually the 'wheels will come off'. You need to be realistic, quite often fitting in training sessions around work and family commitments.

So what positive steps can you take? Firstly it is a lot easier to train with friends or like-minded people. If you are taking on this journey alone, then have a look around. You will be amazed at how many swimming clubs, podcasts, website forums etc there are out there. It can be incredibly comforting to know other people share the same experiences and have the same doubts you may be feeling.

If you can, adopt the buddy system. Training with someone else, even if you are at totally different levels and training differently can still be very motivating. Just to meet up at a set time and discuss how training is going can drag you out of the house when you otherwise might be tempted to skip a session.

There are two things you can always say to yourself when you are having a bad day, feeling tired and thinking of missing a session. Start by fooling your brain by saying to yourself: 'I am just going to do the warm-up'. Once you have got ready and warm, 99 per cent of the time you will feel ready to hit the more intense work. Secondly, constantly remind yourself that training is all about consistency over a period of time. Start to miss too many sessions, that consistency is gone and your body cannot make up the lost time.

Race Day

If you want one word to sum up the state you want your mind to be in on race day then that word is 'positivity'. If you have done the training and your targets are realistic then there is no reason not to be positive.

To help your state of mind on race day there are some basic things you should do. Always prepare the logistics of the day in advance: your kit, travel and accommodation arrangements, and so on, allowing plenty of time so that you have no last-minute panics before the race

There is often a lot of talk and chatter on race days. Keep calm and positive. Many people use the image of 'being in a bubble'. In that bubble you can create your own calm and keep a positive environment.

If you are entering an endurance event the key is not to get ahead

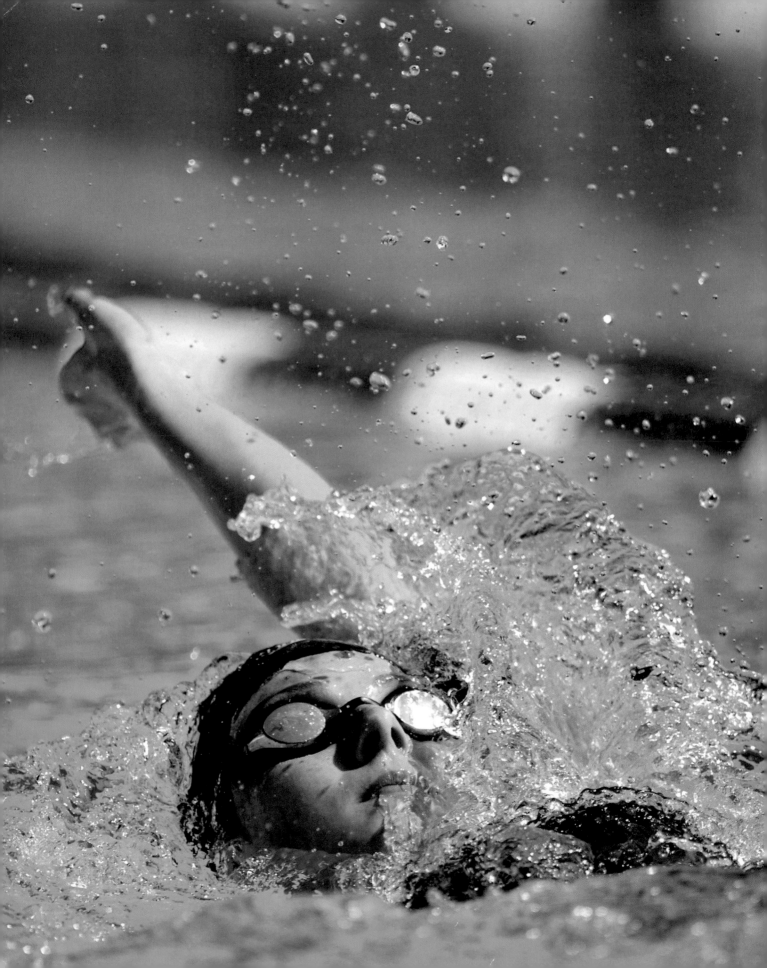

of yourself but to remain with the 'moment'. If you have trained correctly and have a race plan, then stick with the plan. Establish the correct pacing quickly and stay with it. Adrenaline will kick into the body and the temptation is often to push it hard from the start but hold back this temptation and stick with your race plan.

There are different ways to keep your mind in the moment. One is to simply count your strokes. This will focus you on the task at hand and stop your mind racing ahead. In endurance events it is very rare if doubts don't enter your mind so do not be concerned if this happens.

It is at these times that you can bring positive images to your mind. The thought of collecting your medals, bragging rights in your local bar or imagining how impressed your family and friends will be all work. It is a good idea to have thought about these images in advance of the race so you can use them at difficult times.

It may be that you get to a point and just realise that your target is slipping away and you simply cannot achieve it. It is at this point where you have to quickly re-evaluate your target and make the necessary pace changes. This

is harder than it sounds. If you have been very determined to achieve a goal and you feel it slipping away the temptation is to just give up. Don't. Re-evaluate and stay in the moment. You will learn a lot about what you can achieve in these races, and when you have finished you will be glad you kept going.

After the race

After the race give yourself time to enjoy and relax. Take a couple of weeks out to yourself and let your body recover. If this was a long endurance event and you pushed yourself hard then your body and mind will need a bit of space and time to recover. You will have worked hard through the training period, which can be very time consuming, so give yourself this space. This is also a good time to evaluate the race, your training and to set new goals.

Whatever happened in the race make sure you take positives from it. It is all too easy to be hard on yourself and not give yourself the credit you deserve. Even if you didn't achieve your targets or were a long way from them, give yourself credit for getting to the start line in a half-decent shape. Having trained and focused on the race is an achievement in itself.

No matter how the race went, look back and see what improvements you could make in the future. For instance, when it came to your training programme, were you realistic about the amount of training you could fit in? Were your targets realistic, or would you like to do a shorter/longer event? Just remember to take a little time to yourself before taking on the next big challenge.

Injury prevention

Well, the good news for swimmers is that this sport is low impact and therefore often prescribed by doctors, physios and trainers as a low-injury-risk sport. However, as soon as you train a little more competitively, add more lengths at a higher pace and intensity, the problems can start to occur.

Why? Well the simple answer is over-use. Micro-traumas form in the muscles, with the main joint areas at risk being the shoulders and knees. The knees are particularly at risk during breaststroke due to the action the legs take (breaststroke knee). There can also be poor blood supply to the muscles, especially the shoulders. This can cause pain in the shoulders, more correctly known as painful arc or rotator cuff tendonitis.

So how to avoid injury? Firstly remember there is an injury risk with any activity – the more you push your body for results the greater the risk. If you avoided all risk then life would be a little dull, so don't be scared to push your body, as the rewards can be great. What you can do is minimize the risk of injury with a few basic precautions.

Conditioning your body in preparation for the extra intensity can make a massive difference.

Although you cannot truly replicate the movement that your muscles make with weights you can strengthen the muscles that are put under pressure.

As discussed in the cross training section (see pages 82-113), avoid doing weight sessions and heavy pool sessions too close together. Make sure you allow a gap of about 18 hours between any heavy training that you do.

The gap does, of course, depend on how conditioned you already are to start with. If it has been a long time since you have done heavy weight work then your muscles will be traumatized by the tough session and you will need more recovery time. A good option is to do light pool sessions for a couple of days following heavy weights.

One of the biggest ways to help prevent injury is to stick to your training programme. Most programmes will have a gradual increase of laps over time and similar increases of intensity over shorter distances (this will often be interval work).

The theory behind this is usually to gain aerobic and anaerobic increases. We also get great muscular benefits. The muscles

should be just overloaded in order to respond by growing stronger and, of course, this extra strength prevents injury as well as helping you achieve your targets.

Strong technique is very important. You often see swimmers trying to swim fast but creating more of a splash than going anywhere. If they continued with this poor technique over long, intense training sessions, there would be a high risk of injury. Technique has the obvious benefit of more power for less energy, but also allows your body to move smoother and easier. For example, in breaststroke the knee is required to rotate, which is an unnatural way for the knee to move. If the movement is performed incorrectly then the knee will be put under further pressure, creating a higher risk of injury.

The final point to consider is stretching. This is an important part of keeping your body balanced and therefore making it less likely to succumb to injury. Pay particular attention to your stretching programme (see pages 75-81).

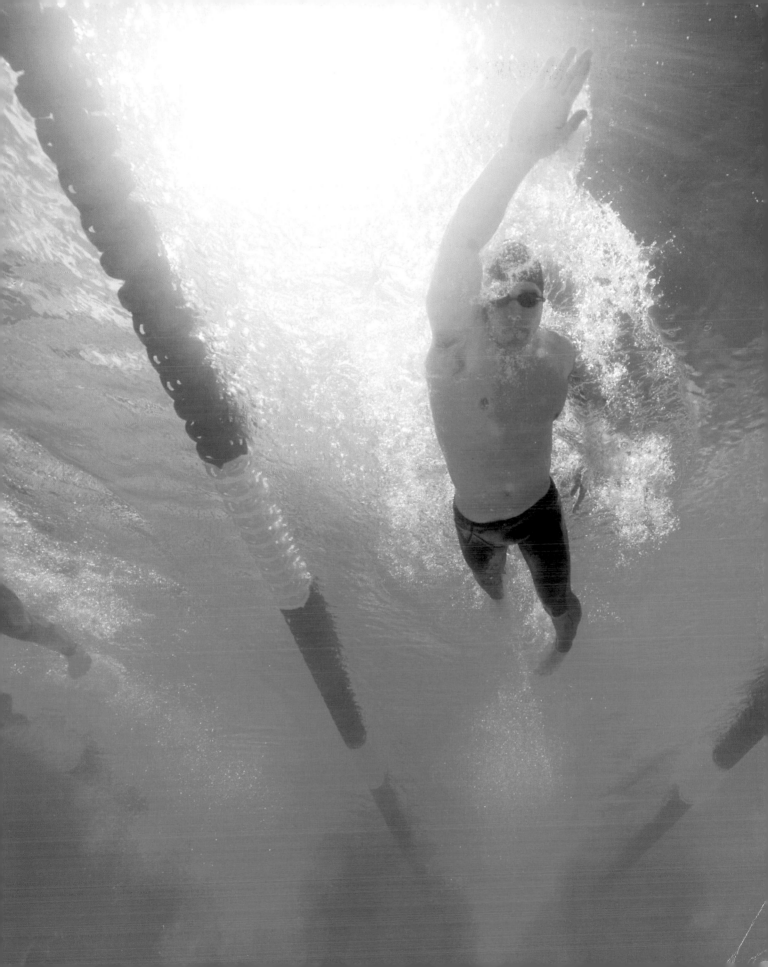

Over-training and over-reaching

The sensation of fatigue is necessary because it lets you know you are pushing your physical limits. You train to improve your performance and your body generally reacts positively to being 'pushed'. However, in certain circumstances, if your body is over-stimulated or stimulated incorrectly, you will suffer adverse effects.

Levels of fatigue

1. The first level of fatigue is hypoglycaemia – the term for abnormally low levels of blood glucose. You reach this when you have exhausted your glycogen stores, haven't ingested enough carbohydrates to produce more blood glucose and are still swimming.

2. Post-training fatigue is the natural response to several hours of intense exercise, which tells you that you are pushing your normal training limits.

3. Over-reaching is the next step up and is when short-term performance drops and develops as a result of an intense training session during a 'high-load' micro-cycle (see page 149). Symptoms are those of normal fatigue. The right amount of recovery will allow you to become faster and stronger. It is, however, a warning.

4. Over-training is the debilitating and long-term (often lasting weeks and sometimes months) fatigue, which degrades rather than stimulates performance.

Overtraining in volume and/or intensity can lead to some inevitable outcomes. Firstly, if you train too hard or over-train, your immune system will be very low, leaving you susceptible to illness. A cold can set you back a long way in your preparation. You would be amazed at what lengths top endurance athletes go to avoid illness.

The other potential problem you face is injury. Over-use of your muscles in the gym or in the pool, where you are repeating the same action over and over again, can lead to those all too familiar injury problems for swimmers, around the shoulders and the knees.

Burnout is also another key issue to consider. If you keep pushing your body as hard as you can in every session for as long as you can you will eventually find yourself not wanting to go to the pool and train. Having a different target for each session will help you get to the side of the pool mentally prepared.

How to prevent over-training

The most frequent causes of over-training are: excessive increase in training loads, insufficient recovery periods, poor diet (insufficient quantity of carbohydrates or other nutritional elements), travel factors and a lack of variety in your training.

So how do you prevent over-training? You need a balance between training and recovery both at long term (mesocycle) and short term (microcycle) (see page 149). This means that after a few weeks of heavy training, the intensity should be reduced for a period of time (usually a week) and the number of rest days should be increased. The purpose of this recovery week is to allow your body complete regeneration.

Most training programmes include one or two rest days per week as well as a day or two of easy swimming, allowing you to recover. Unvaried training programmes without alternating periods of high and low volume/intensity also severely increase the risk of over-training. The key is planning your own personal training programme to occasionally over-reach but not over-train. Your challenge is finding your own individual boundary.

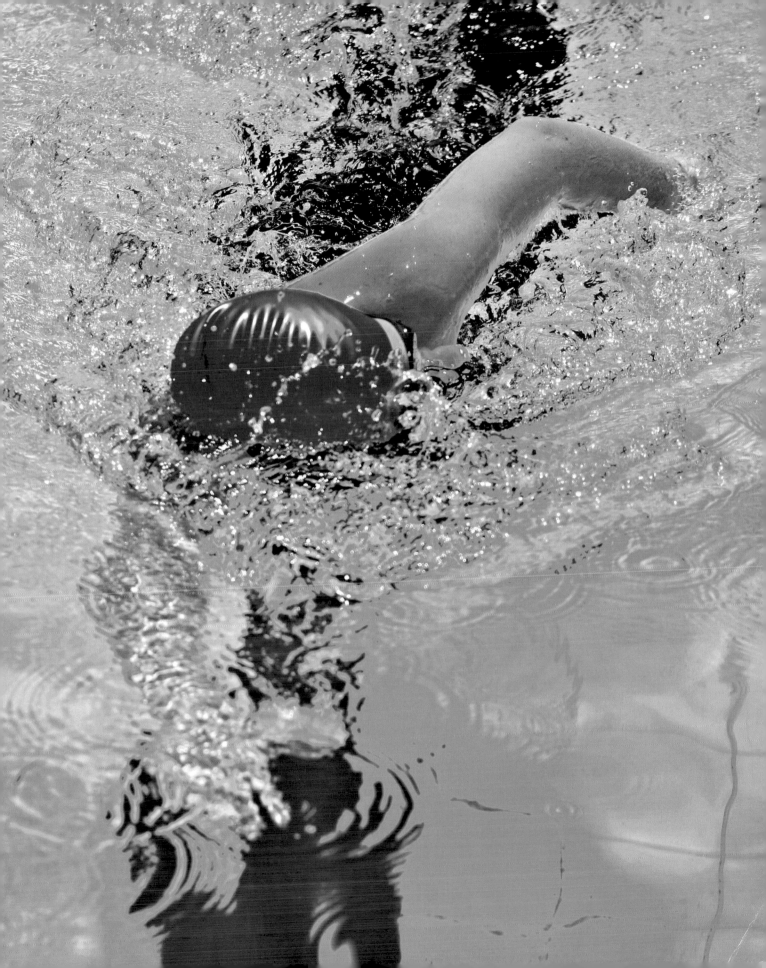

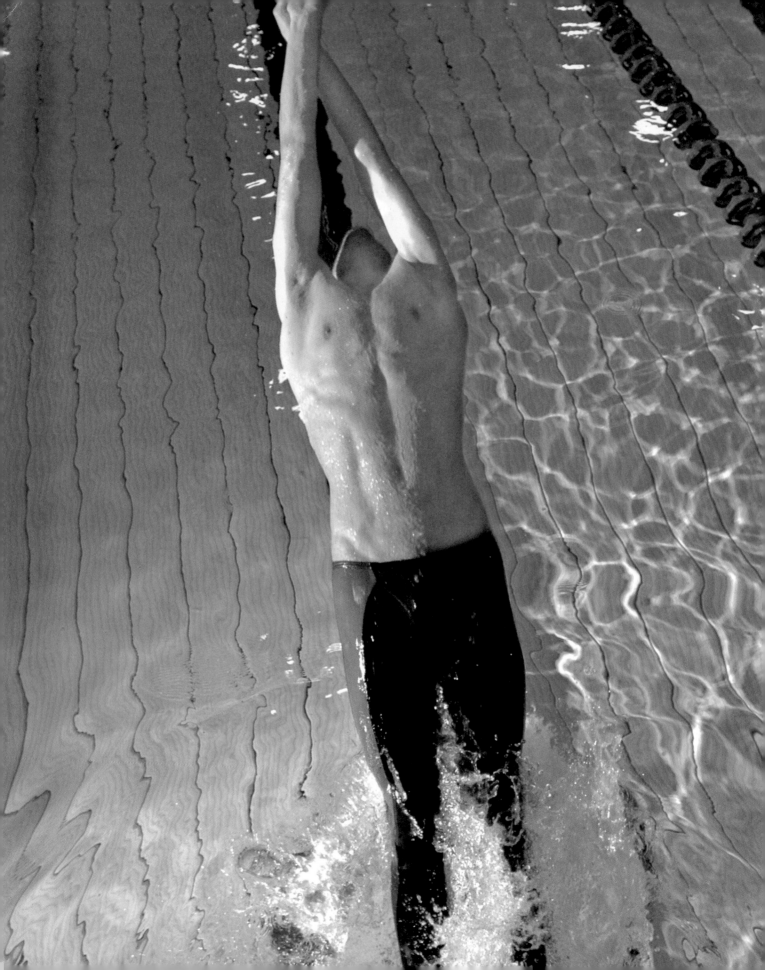

Stretches

Stretching plays a crucial role in injury prevention and enhancing overall athletic performance and yet it is often overlooked and neglected by many athletes as the 'soft' part of the training programme. Stretching is every bit as important as pushing a big, heavy weight or putting in those extra high-intensity kilometres in your training. Don't miss your stretching regime just to get in a few more minutes hard training. It's the wrong move.

By training regularly you will be shortening certain muscles. To ensure you maintain an equal muscular balance throughout your body it is imperative you do not skip the stretches that help to keep these muscles in shape. Although it is important to stretch before a session to prepare for what is to follow, it is also vital to stretch afterwards as well.

This can be hard to do after a tough session or race but generally athletes should spend a lot longer stretching after a heavy training session than before it. In general, it is best to do your stretching at the end of a workout, stretching out the muscles you have just worked for a minimum of one minute each. This will help prevent the shortening of muscles and muscular imbalances in your body, which can cause pain, injury and may also stop you from training or competing.

So, for example, if you have performed a set of squats you will need to stretch your quads, hamstrings, glutes, calves and lower back. This is just basic maintenance stretching. When you start to clock up more kilometres in training it is advisable to use your rest days to take deeper and longer stretches. Many people neglect this area of their training. A day off is a day off a lot of us think. But get into the habit of giving those muscles you have worked so hard during the week, a really good stretch. You can also do your maintenance stretches on your rest breaks when training.

For the deeper stretches, which really improve your flexibility and balance, it's advisable to find a suitable yoga or stretch class. Stretching really can make a difference between achieving your goals and failing to get to the start line. Take it seriously, do not think it's just something you need to get out of the way before the serious work: this is part of the serious work.

Consider also that before a training session or important race your stress levels can rise, so before stretching you should consider paying attention to what most of us take for granted: breathing. Slowly take a couple of long breaths in and out through your nose. Or take one big, deep breath from your stomach. In sport, especially at the highest level, small details can make a significant difference. That's why even a tiny relief from your stress might result in finding just that energy you need even if it's just for a few seconds to help keep you focused and relaxed.

Over the next few pages you will see details of some key stretches. You can use these before and after training/racing but do not neglect to do these stretches on your day off. Also, while these are key stretches for many of the muscles you will use, do not rely on these entirely. Remember to stretch out as many muscles as possible to keep muscular balance.

Stretches – quads

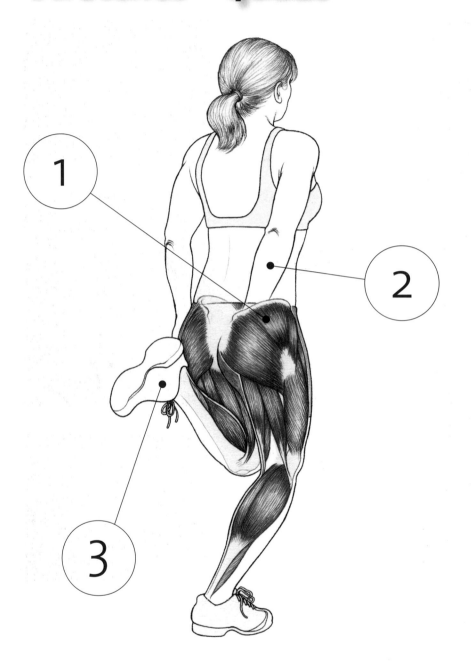

1 Stand tall, take the front of the foot (shoelaces) and bring heel into your backside and pull gently until you feel the quad pulling. For a deeper stretch push your working hip forward.

2 If you struggle with balance simply hold onto something with your other hand. Before races and training sessions hold each leg for 10-20 seconds, one time on each leg.

3 For a dynamic stretch, once your quads are warm you can kick your heels into your backside 10-15 times without using your hands. Obviously, if you want to do the dynamic stretch you will need a dry surface – don't do this by a wet pool.

MUSCLES STRETCHED   *QUADS AND HIP FLEXES*

Stretches – arm swings

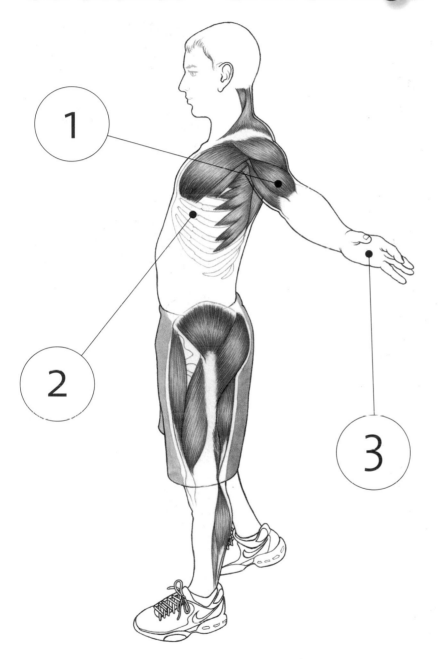

1 Stand tall and circle your arms in a windmill fashion four to six times forwards and four to six times backwards. Start slowly and build momentum gradually as you complete the swings.

2 Follow this with an arm swing to stretch out your chest. Start with your arms together pointing forwards and then gently swing them out to your side keeping them horizontal. Keep it smooth and avoid a fast, jerky movement as this puts too much pressure on your muscles.

3 To finish, now your muscles are loose, clasp you hands together behind your back just below the base of your spine. Gently lift arms up and away from your body to stretch out your chest.

MUSCLES STRETCHED *DELTOIDS AND CHEST*

Stretches – shoulder opener

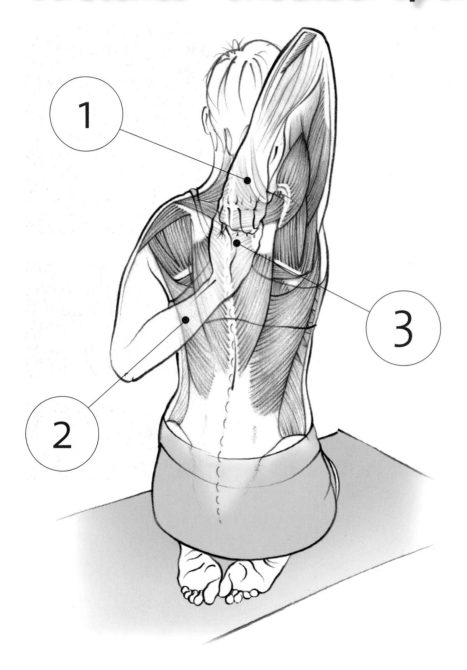

1 This stretch can be done either standing or sitting down. Point one arm towards the ceiling, brushing against your ear. Drop your hand down as far as possible to the centre of your back. Push other hand up your back and aim to clasp them together. This takes some flexibility and practice.

2 If you cannot bring your two hands together to meet, hold a towel in the top hand and clasp the towel with your lower hand. Gently pull evenly with both arms on the towel to stretch.

3 Hold the stretch for 15-20 seconds and remember to stretch both sides.

MUSCLES STRETCHED   *SHOULDERS, DELTOIDS AND TRICEPS*

Stretches – triceps

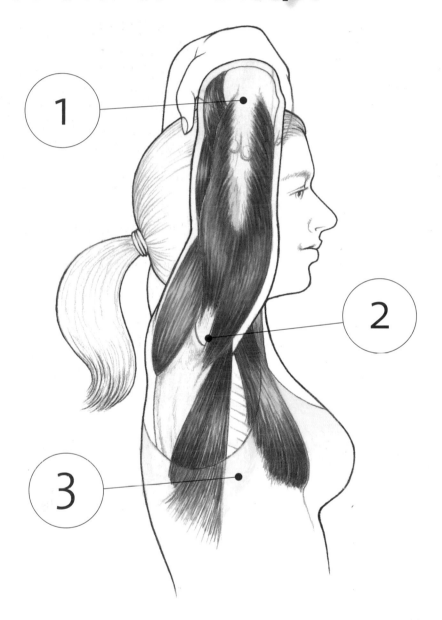

1 This stretch can be done either standing or sitting down. Your starting position is to reach towards the ceiling with one arm and drop the arm across your head. Using your other hand gently push that arm further behind your head until you feel your tricep stretching.

2 To increase the intensity and add a side stretch at the same time lean sideways away from the working arm by a few degrees and hold.

3 Hold the stretch for 15-20 seconds and remember to stretch both sides.

MUSCLES STRETCHED   *TRICEPS AND LATERALS*

Stretches – hamstring

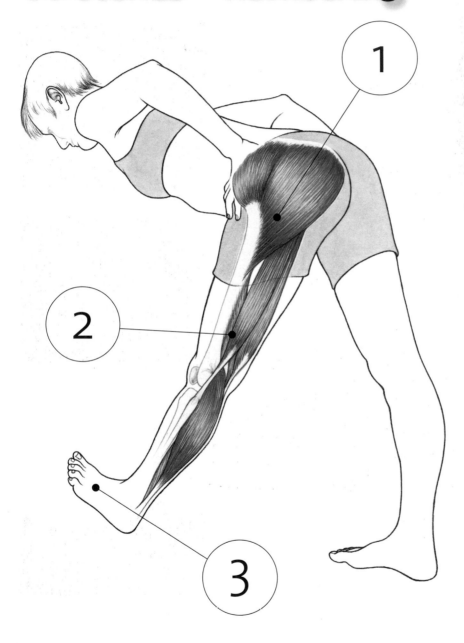

1 For your starting position stretch one leg out forwards in a natural step. Place your hands on your hips. Then lean forwards at the waist keeping your back straight and long until you feel the hamstring stretch.

2 Hold stretch for 30 seconds, relax for 10 seconds then repeat, increasing the range of the stretch this time and hold for a further 30 seconds. Repeat on other hamstring.

3 To add a calf stretch at the same time, lift up your toes to flex your front foot.

MUSCLES STRETCHED *HAMSTRINGS AND CALVES*

Stretches – seated adductor

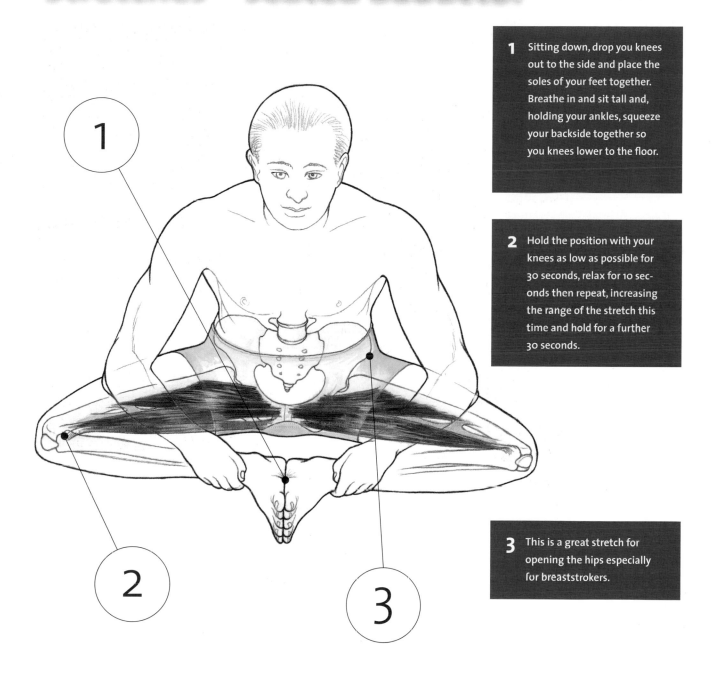

1 Sitting down, drop you knees out to the side and place the soles of your feet together. Breathe in and sit tall and, holding your ankles, squeeze your backside together so you knees lower to the floor.

2 Hold the position with your knees as low as possible for 30 seconds, relax for 10 seconds then repeat, increasing the range of the stretch this time and hold for a further 30 seconds.

3 This is a great stretch for opening the hips especially for breaststrokers.

MUSCLES STRETCHED   *ADDUCTORS*

cross training

// STRONGER // TOUGHER
// MORE POWERFUL

The basics

If you are training for a particular sport there is no question that the best way to get fit for that purpose is to actually do that sport. If you want to be a swimmer then swim, swim and swim some more, it's as simple as that.

So why cross train then?

Here we focus on four reasons to cross train: strengthening a weakness in a particular muscle or muscle group, injury prevention, motivation and ensuring that you maintain your general fitness.

Most coaches will include a strength-training programme into an athlete's schedule whatever sport they are involved in. The amount of work that needs to be done in the gym can vary from sport to sport and, of course, the distance you are training for and the specific goals you have.

Generally, the shorter events will require more power and strength, which can be gained with weights. For endurance events it is advisable that the strength training is done well away from the heavy pool work. For example, if you are considering entering an event in six months, start your gym work with heavy weights and low reps (eight to 12 reps) for six to eight weeks, then lower the weights but increase the reps (maximum 15) for a couple of weeks. After this you can then start to eliminate all weight work and concentrate on your swimming.

However, everything depends on how serious and challenging your targets are. You can keep working on the strength training after these guidelines but be aware that your swimming could suffer as muscle fatigue may prevent you training properly for your main event. If you don't want to give up your cross training completely you could substitute this gym work for increased core work or specific stretching exercises. Overall, then, the benefits of spending time in the gym will be extra power in the pool, but don't overdo it – your training should also keep your core goals in mind.

Identify and strengthen weaknesses in the chain

One benefit of cross training is targeting a particular weakness in your body that is holding your swimming back. Once you have identified that weakness in your body while swimming you can head to the gym and really focus on that particular area, whether it's your legs, your shoulders or simply building up muscle groups for general body balance. So, for example, if you find some weakness in your hamstrings (back of the leg) and glutes (backside) while swimming you can use the squats (see page 88) and hamstring curls (see page 90) to strengthen these areas. By focussing on these muscles in the gym you really will notice a difference when you are in the pool.

However, it must still be remembered at all times that a lot of the pain we experience is due to the build up of lactic acid and the best way to combat this is to train in your chosen sport to keep the essential muscles for swimming in active use.

Injury prevention

Prevention of injury is probably the main reason to do specific training for your sport. Injuries can ruin months of hard work and for us non-sporting professionals, as well as ruining the sporting dream, this can make daily life very uncomfortable – just ask anyone with bad back pain they picked up in sport who has to sit in an office for eight hours a day.

When increasing your training workload in the pool you may experience discomfort in your body, as muscles are asked to perform tasks at a much higher level to anything they have known before.

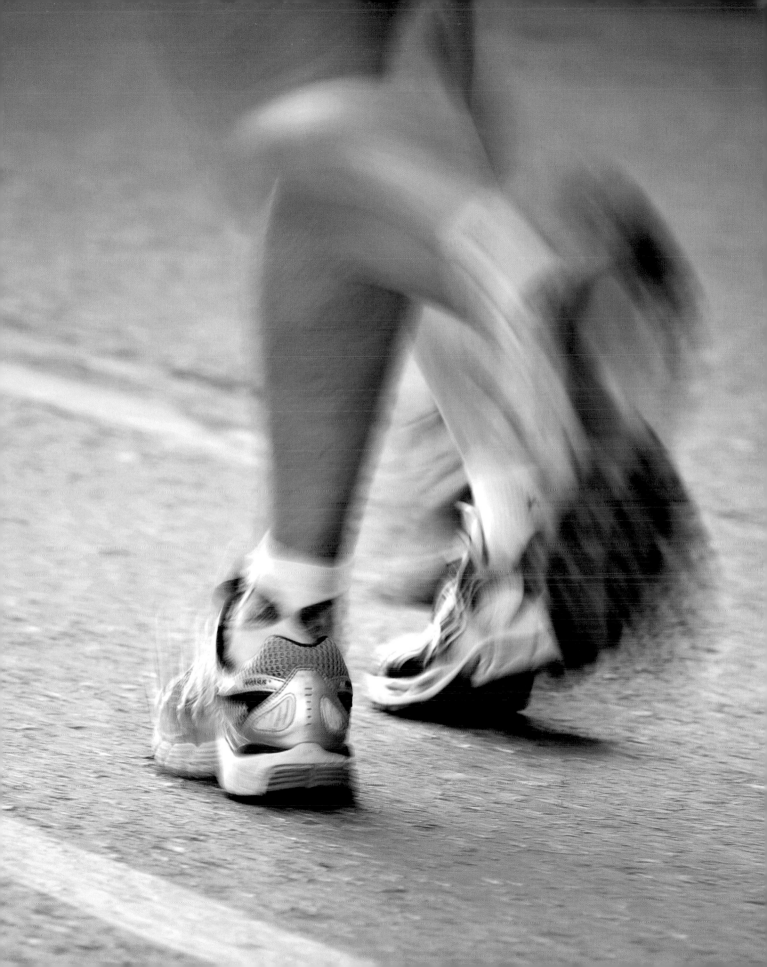

For example, if your hamstrings become very strong and tight and your opposite muscles (the quads) are weak then this can cause the pelvis to be held in a tilted alignment, which in turn causes poor back alignment and back pain.

For these reasons, in the strength programmes outlined (see pages 111-113) you will find exercises which are not only geared towards swimming, but will also help keep a good muscular balance in your body. In the core section you will also find some Pilates exercises.

These exercises are slightly modified for ease of use. However, if you can attend some Pilates or yoga classes these are an excellent way of keeping your core strong, maintaining an equal muscle balance and keeping your muscles supple. The added benefit of these exercises is that as these exercises are low impact there is a reduced risk of injury and because of the

low-energy output they can even be done on your rest day.

Stretching regularly also plays a key role in injury prevention and this aspect of your training should not be ignored (See Fitness & Training pages 75-81).

Motivation
Sometimes, when training for a specific event, you will just need a break from the routine of pounding the laps in the pool. By having one day a week where you train your body in a different way you can really freshen up your mind as well. It can also be a good idea to add in some basic targets for your resistance training to keep motivated. You could, for instance, aim to increase your weight load by a certain percentage over a two-month period.

Be aware that the targets you set will very much depend on where your starting point is. If you are

already experienced in strength training your gains will be small because you will already have reached a decent level, so be realistic when setting goals.

General fitness
Many people start on their swimming journey as a way of getting into shape and this is one of the greatest benefits of the sport. However, you must remember that if you just train in the sport you will only be fit for this sport. A certain amount of fitness will cross over to other fitness areas, but to keep yourself healthy and looking good often requires something a bit more specific. This can be seen clearly in different running distances. A good 100-metre runner will often struggle to do a good marathon time and vice-versa. So if one of your goals from swimming is good overall health you should not ignore cross training.

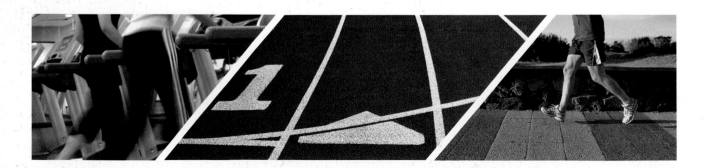

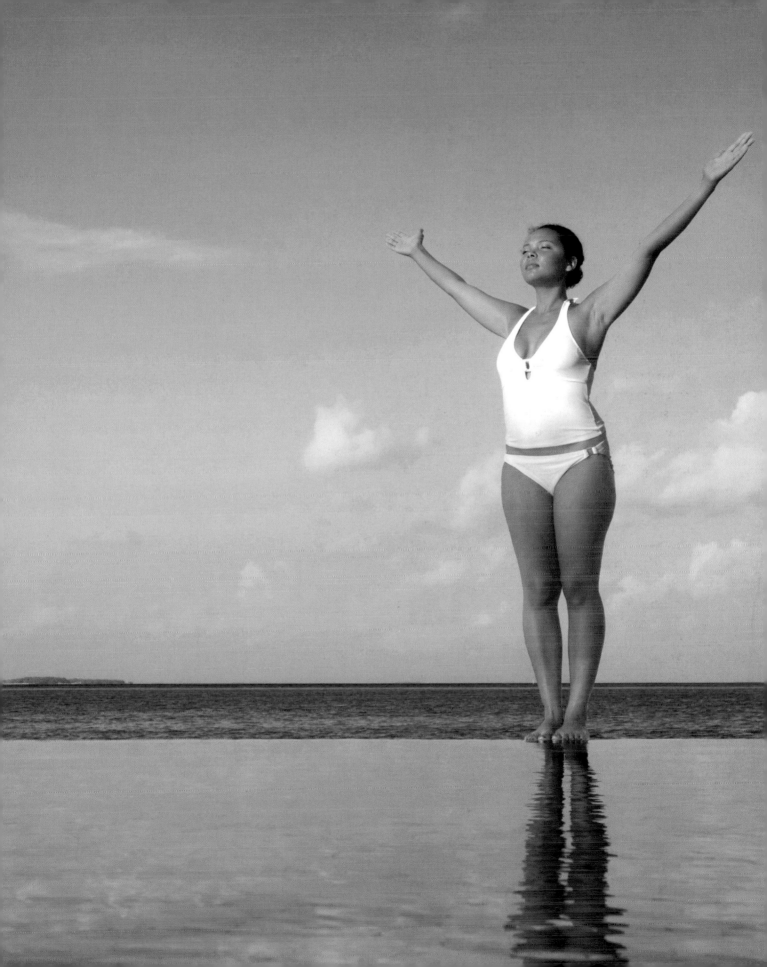

Legs – squats

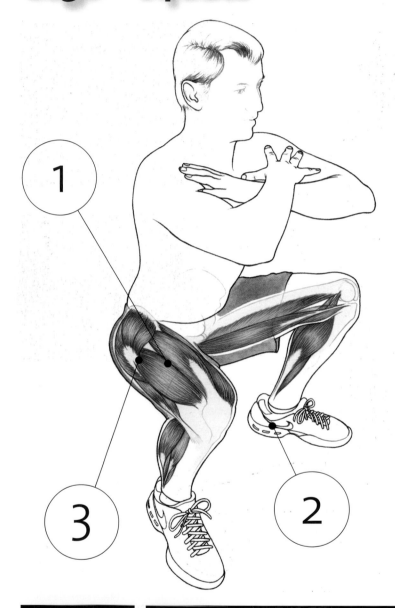

1 Keep knees soft and gently squeeze abs and bum. Tip your hips back as if you are sitting down in a chair, then go down until your upper leg is parallel with the floor. Push back up to the start position.

2 Keep all the weight driving through your heels, as this will maximize the workload in the glutes and hamstrings. Make sure your back stays long and keep knees over your middle toes.

3 As you start to fatigue, focus on keeping your abs and bum muscles engaged as this will protect the lower back. Use your breath to help, releasing breath as you press up.

Muscles Used	How will it improve my swimming?
Primary: quads, glutes, hamstrings, lower back (erector spinae). Secondary: calves.	Knee injuries are the curse of swimmers. This drill will strengthen the muscle groups around the joint and help you to avoid ligament damage as well as adding the all-important explosive power needed in the pool.

Legs – lunges

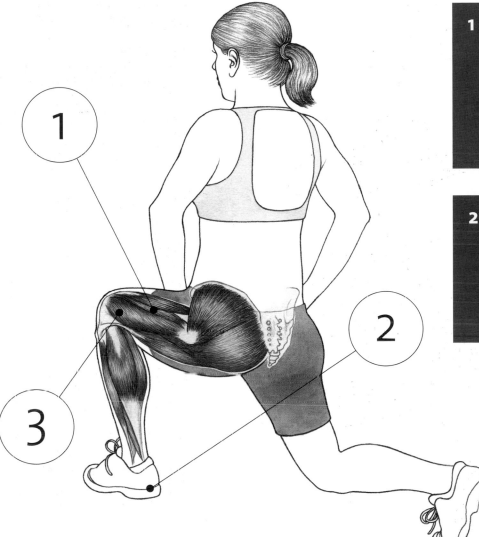

1 With feet hip-width apart keep knees soft and body tall, then take a long step back keeping back heel off the floor. Aim your back knee down to the floor and keep the front knee in line with your middle toe.

2 You need to keep your weight pressing through the front heel without allowing the front knee to travel forwards. Keep your pelvis gently tucked under your body.

3 The feel of the lunge movement is straight down and up. There should be no forward movement. This will keep the pressure on the front knee.

Muscles Used

Primary: quads, glutes, hamstrings, calves.

How will it improve my swimming?

Breaststrokers use these muscles on the kick stroke and this exercise will help you gain more power and efficiency. Maintaining the tone of the muscle group will help avoid pulls and strains from this unnatural motion.

Legs – hamstring curls

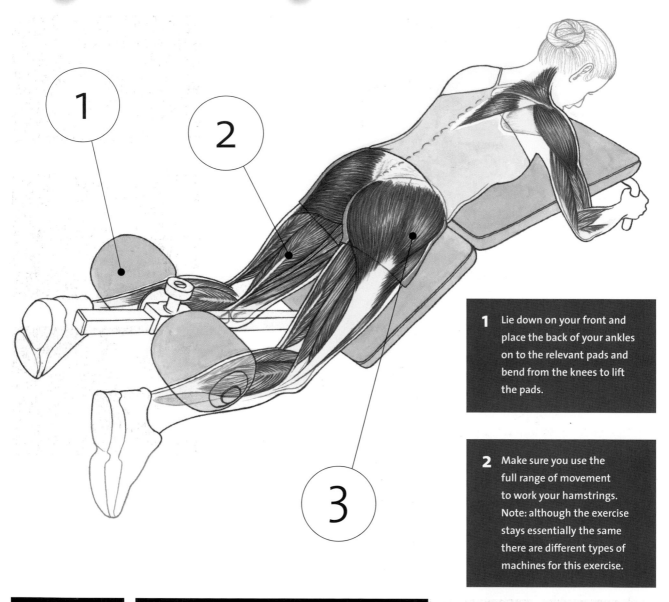

1 Lie down on your front and place the back of your ankles on to the relevant pads and bend from the knees to lift the pads.

2 Make sure you use the full range of movement to work your hamstrings. Note: although the exercise stays essentially the same there are different types of machines for this exercise.

3 Avoid allowing your hips to move up and down. Keep your hips still by pulling in your abs. This will help also help to avoid back injuries.

Muscles Used	How will it improve my swimming?
Primary: hamstrings, glutes.	Most of the momentum in freestyle and butterfly comes from your backside. This exercise builds the most important part of your swimming engine up as well as keeping the rest of the leg muscles in shape.

Legs – bench steps

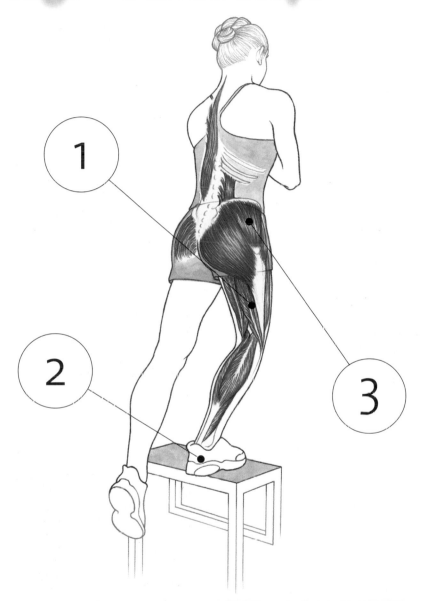

1. Stand about 30cm (about 12 inches) away from a step or bench. Step one foot up before bringing the other leg up, always keeping the foot and knee at a right angle.

2. When stepping onto the bench with your first leg, carefully put the heel down first. This will keep your body secure on the bench and activate the correct muscles.

3. Always keep the body straight and tall. The temptation is to lean forward from the hips. To increase the intensity you can hold weights in each hand.

Muscles Used	How will it improve my swimming?
Primary: Quads, glutes. Secondary: hamstrings, calves.	The stronger your calves and quadriceps are the more balance you will have on the blocks. The more power these muscles can generate at the gun, the bigger the advantage you will gain over your rivals.

Legs – calf raises

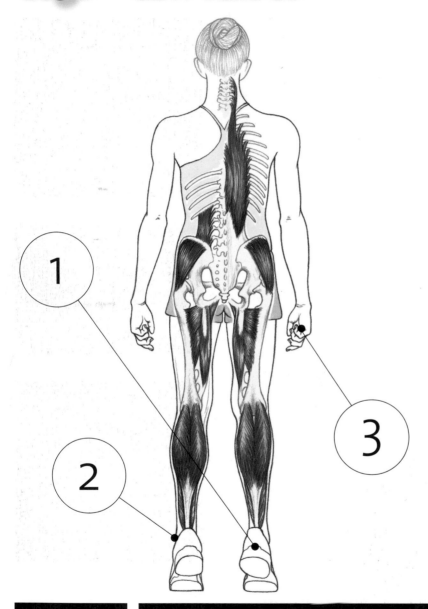

1 Keep feet hip-width apart and your body tall, then rise up high onto the balls of the feet, and lower back to starting position.

2 Keep your ankles in neutral alignment. The temptation is to let your heels fall out to the side. Always keep the whole body lifted and straight.

3 To increase the intensity you can hold a weight in each hand. If no equipment is available simply use cans of food or something heavy and easy to hold.

Muscles Used	How will it improve my swimming?
Primary: calves.	This drill works the calves, which are vital for maximizing spring from the start, especially in backstroke where you start off the wall. It may not look very taxing but you will soon see the benefits on the clock.

Legs – jump squats

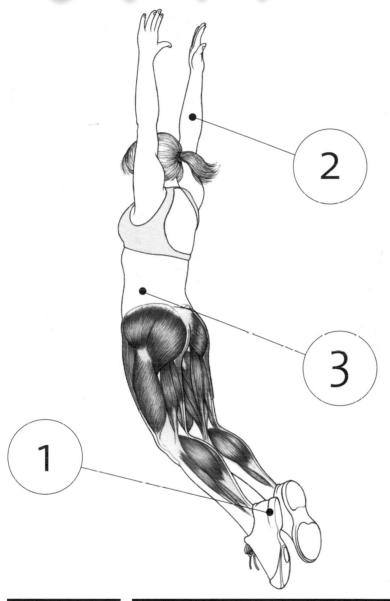

1 This is advanced dynamic work. Take a shallow squat then jump forward pushing equally off both feet to jump as far as you can. Land through a heel-to-toe action and bend the knees on impact to cushion the landing.

2 Take a pause between each rep to steady the body so you are in a strong starting position. You can use your arms to gain momentum, using a natural swing.

3 As with all dynamic work there is a high risk of injury if the exercise is not performed correctly, so as you get tired make sure your abs are gently squeezed in and landings are soft. If you can't maintain this then it's time to stop.

Muscles Used	How will it improve my swimming?
Primary: quads, glutes, hamstrings, lower back. Secondary: calves.	Your legs contribute more to your overall power than your arms and this exercise maintains all the muscles groups in the lower limbs that are vital in every stroke and start.

Shoulders – shoulder press

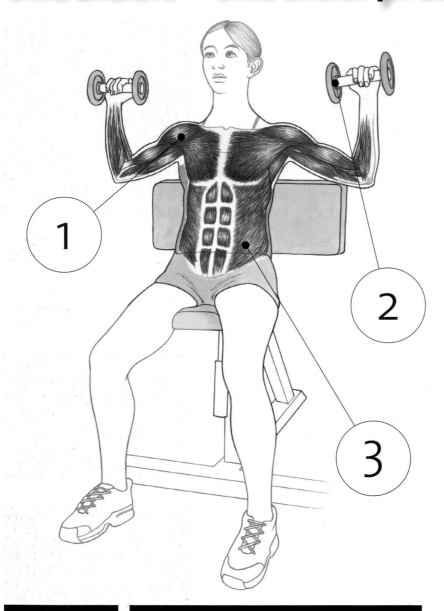

1 Sitting down, ensure elbows are at shoulder height with arms at a right angle and the hands and weight heading up. Push the weights up to the ceiling, and gently bring them together at the top.

2 The weights will move in a slight arc, but keep control and don't allow them to bang into each other at the top.

3 Be very aware of the lower back in this exercise. Do not allow the back to arch. You can combat this by squeezing your abs and gently tucking the pelvis under.

Muscles Used

Primary: shoulders (deltoids).
Secondary: triceps.

How will it improve my swimming?

Along with knee problems, shoulder injuries are the main bugbear for swimmers as it is the most worked joint in the body in freestyle, butterfly and backstroke. This exercise will help keep them strong.

* To do this exercise without weights, start in the same position but put both feet on a resistance band and pull round in an arc from your shoulders in the same path to the top as with weights.

Shoulders – lateral raises

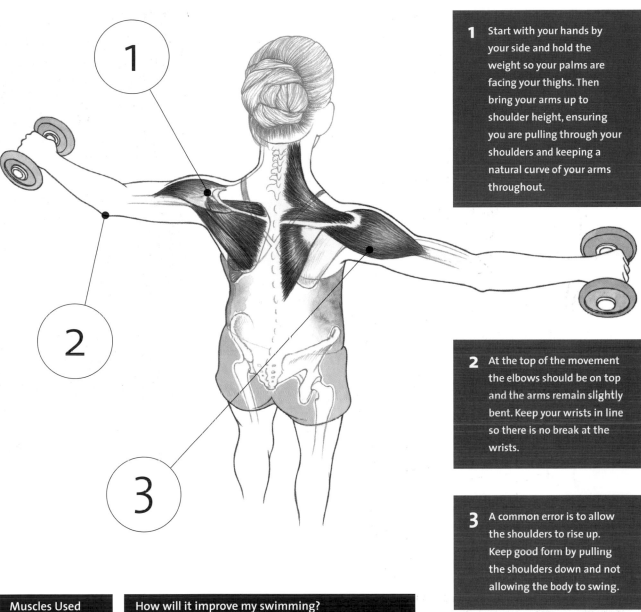

1 Start with your hands by your side and hold the weight so your palms are facing your thighs. Then bring your arms up to shoulder height, ensuring you are pulling through your shoulders and keeping a natural curve of your arms throughout.

2 At the top of the movement the elbows should be on top and the arms remain slightly bent. Keep your wrists in line so there is no break at the wrists.

3 A common error is to allow the shoulders to rise up. Keep good form by pulling the shoulders down and not allowing the body to swing.

* To do this exercise without weights, start in the same position but put both feet on a resistance band and pull round in an arc from your shoulders in the same path to the top as with weights.

Muscles Used	How will it improve my swimming?
Primary: shoulders (deltoids).	Throwing your arms back is an important part of the backstroke start – this exercise will build the muscles needed for a powerful stretch as you leave the wall to complement your kick off.

Shoulders – rotator cuff

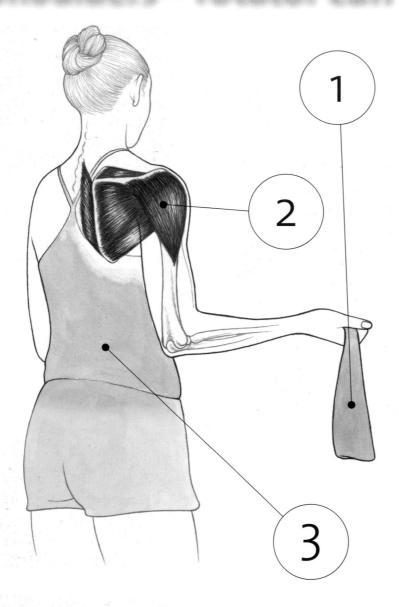

1 Using a resistance band, start with one end of the band tied to a pole and hold the other end in one hand. Ensuring you keep your working elbow close to your body pull your hand across the body at a right angle.

2 While keeping your elbow at a right angle, open your arm outwards from your body so you are squeezing the back of your shoulder.

3 This is a great exercise for keeping the shoulder alignment open. Make sure your posture stays true so you don't allow any movement around your back.

Muscles Used	How will it improve my swimming?
Primary: back of shoulder (rotator cuff).	Backstroke and freestyle place a heavy strain on your rotator cuff muscles and they are commonly pulled or damaged. This drill keeps them in shape for the rigours of the two fastest strokes.

Shoulders – dumb-bell raises

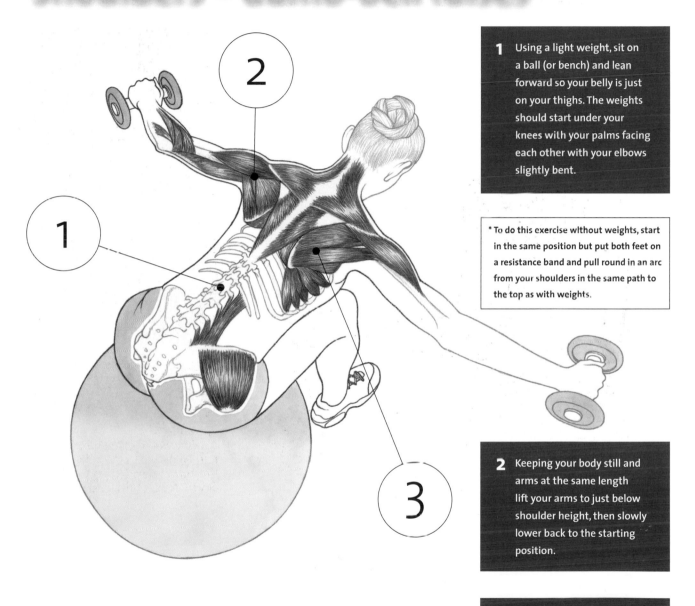

1 Using a light weight, sit on a ball (or bench) and lean forward so your belly is just on your thighs. The weights should start under your knees with your palms facing each other with your elbows slightly bent.

* To do this exercise without weights, start in the same position but put both feet on a resistance band and pull round in an arc from your shoulders in the same path to the top as with weights.

2 Keeping your body still and arms at the same length lift your arms to just below shoulder height, then slowly lower back to the starting position.

3 Although your body is bent over, remember to keep your abs working and keep breathing. Avoid lifting your shoulders as this means you will be pulling down from the shoulder.

Muscles Used	How will it improve my swimming?
Primary: rear (posterior), shoulders (deltoids).	Clearing the water with your arms is crucial in the arm stroke. This exercise will help prevent fatigue in the shoulders, which leads to a lower, less-efficient stroke at the end of races.

Shoulders – bent-over rowing

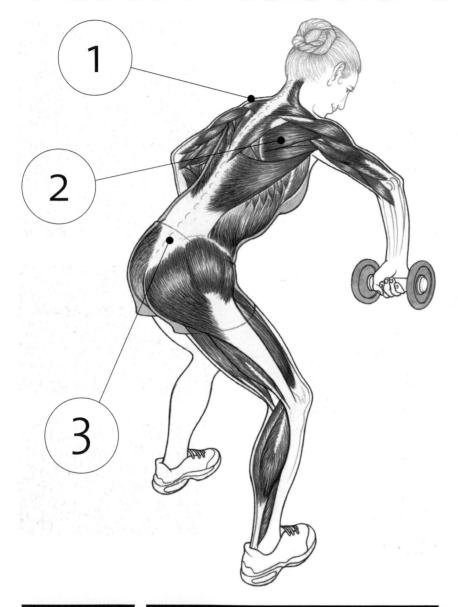

1 Start with the weights down by your knees. Stay in this bent over position and squeeze the weights in towards the belly button in a rowing movement, before straightening your arms to the starting position again.

2 When lifting the weights feel your shoulder blades squeezing together. This will concentrate the workload in the centre of your back.

3 Staying in this position can be tough on your lower back and there is a temptation to curve your lower spine outwards. Avoid this by keeping your pelvis in the correct alignment and squeezing your abs.

Muscles Used	How will it improve my swimming?
Primary: neck, shoulder and back (trapezius). Secondary: biceps.	This drill helps with the important rolling of the shoulders in backstroke as well as strengthening the muscles around the joint, which is so important in all strokes. It also helps to protect against injury.

* To do this exercise without weights, start in the same position but put both feet on a resistance band and pull round in an arc from your shoulders in the same path to the top as with weights.

Back – dead lift

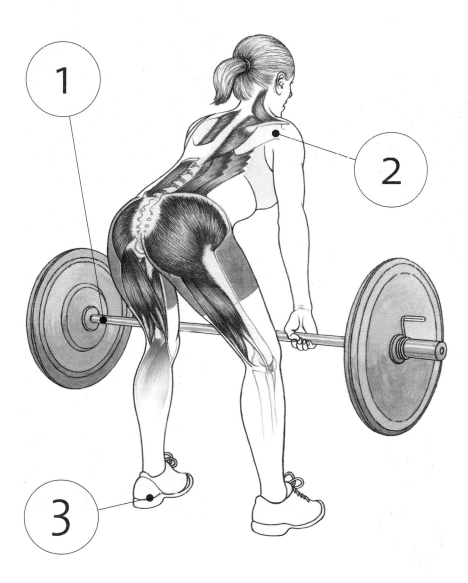

1 Start with your heels under your hips, legs slightly bent, your back straight, hands just wider than your thighs and palms facing the body. Then lower the bar down to your knees by leaning forwards and concentrating on working your back. Pause briefly and come back to your starting point.

2 As you go through the reps keep your back long and do not allow any flexion or extension from your knees. Shoulders should be pulled back at all times.

3 All the weight should be in the heel of your foot and your knees soft without bending them. Avoid doing squats.

Muscles Used	How will it improve my swimming?
Primary: lower back, hamstrings, glutes.	An important drill to maintain strength in your lower back and backside. It helps to keep your hips up in backstroke.

Back – prone back extension

1 Lie on your belly button on a ball with your feet shoulder width apart and place your finger tips lightly on your chest (or the back of your head). Gently lift your upper body upwards then lower to the starting position.

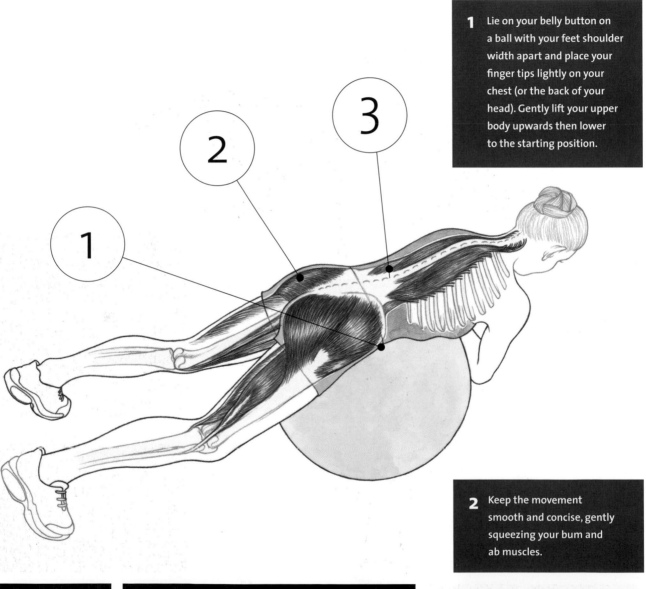

2 Keep the movement smooth and concise, gently squeezing your bum and ab muscles.

Muscles Used	How will it improve my swimming?
Primary: lower back.	There is nothing more painful than a bad back and this drill, using a gym ball, helps to maintain strength in the muscles that support your spine as well as working major groups that contribute to a powerful foot kick.

3 Rolling further forward on the ball can make the exercise more intense but be careful as this can put more pressure on the lower back.

Chest – lateral pull down

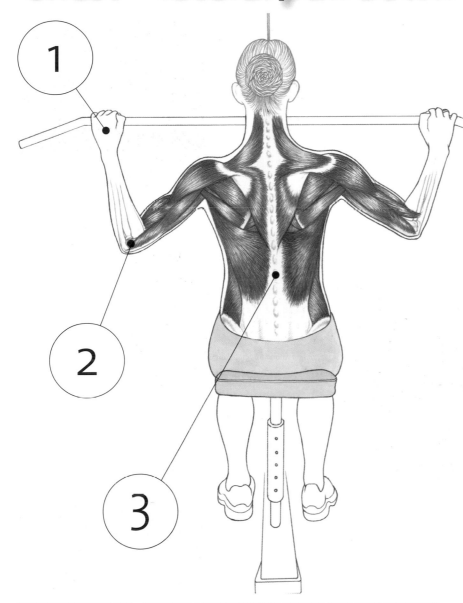

1 Hands should be positioned one and a half times of your shoulder width apart. Keep your body tall and lean back slightly. Pull the bar down towards the upper chest and keep control and then release back to the starting position.

2 Feel your elbows as you pull down, as this will activate your back muscles. Keep your hands light on the bar – if you grip too hard your fore-arms will fatigue quickly.

3 As your body fatigues avoid allowing your back to swing and your bum to come off the seat. Also avoid pulling down quickly.

Muscles Used	How will it improve my swimming?
Primary: laterals. Secondary: biceps.	An important muscles group when your arms are in the water on the pull stroke in butterfly and freestyle. The more power you can generate from here, the more water you can move to propel yourself forward.

Chest – press-ups

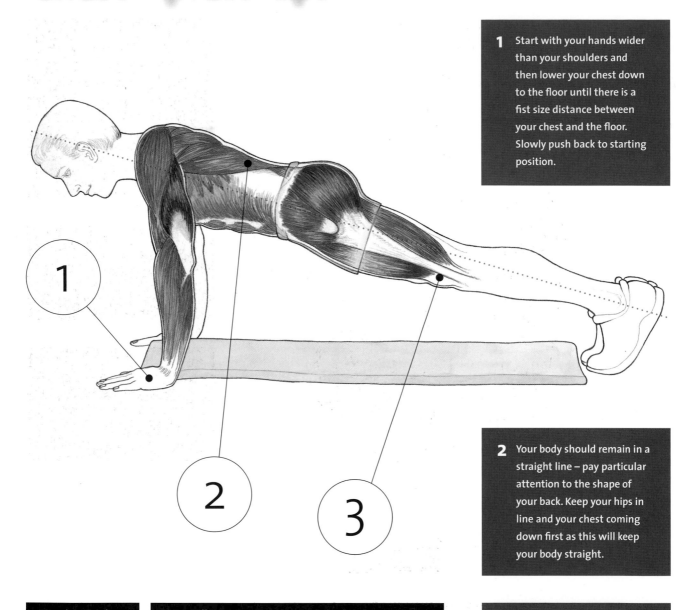

1 Start with your hands wider than your shoulders and then lower your chest down to the floor until there is a fist size distance between your chest and the floor. Slowly push back to starting position.

2 Your body should remain in a straight line – pay particular attention to the shape of your back. Keep your hips in line and your chest coming down first as this will keep your body straight.

3 You can lower your knees down to lower the intensity of the press-up. You should also do this if you feel you are losing your body alignment.

Muscles Used

Primary: pecs.
Secondary: triceps.

How will it improve my swimming?

It is important not to get bottom heavy as a swimmer. Press-ups will help you to keep the balance in power and weight between the two halves of your body and equilibrium in the water.

Arms – bicep curls

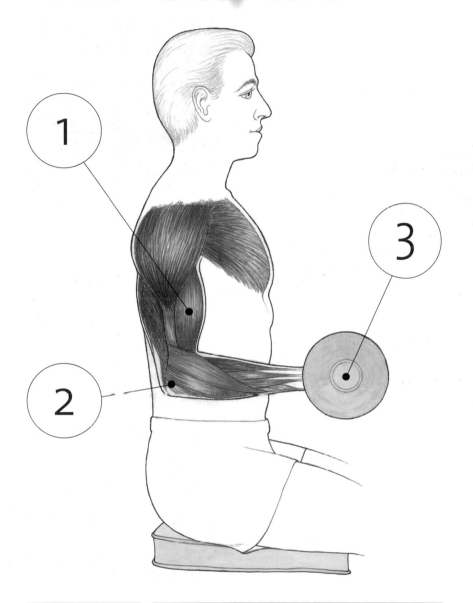

1 Hold the weights with your palms facing forwards while keeping your hands at a natural carrying grip. Bend at the elbow and curl the weights to your chest. Pause briefly then curl back to the horizontal starting position.

2 Keep your elbows close to your body and do not allow them to pull back behind the body alignment.

3 Your hands need to remain strong but soft. If you grip too hard you will feel your forearms work more as opposed to your biceps.

Muscles Used	How will it improve my swimming?
Primary: biceps.	You are not trying to look like Charles Atlas so don't overdo this one – look for tone not size. This exercise helps you to improve power in the upper arm, which is important across all four strokes.

* To do this exercise without weights, start in the same position but put both feet on a resistance band and pull round in an arc from your shoulders in the same path to the top as with weights.

Arms – tricep dips

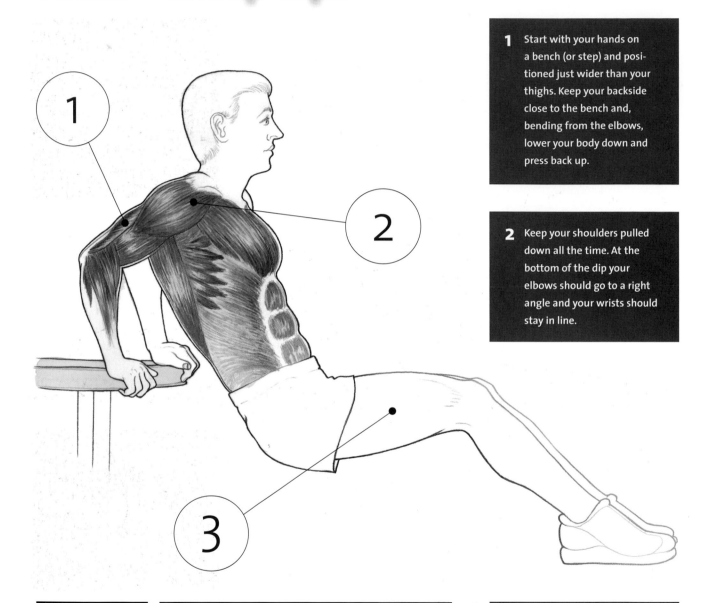

1 Start with your hands on a bench (or step) and positioned just wider than your thighs. Keep your backside close to the bench and, bending from the elbows, lower your body down and press back up.

2 Keep your shoulders pulled down all the time. At the bottom of the dip your elbows should go to a right angle and your wrists should stay in line.

3 You can make this exercise more intense by straightening your legs and flexing your feet. When doing this keep your backside close to your body.

Muscles Used	How will it improve my swimming?
Primary: triceps.	Triceps play a major role in the pull stroke in breaststroke and by toning them up you will make yourself more efficient. This also works some of the chest muscles to maintain tone.

Core – front plank

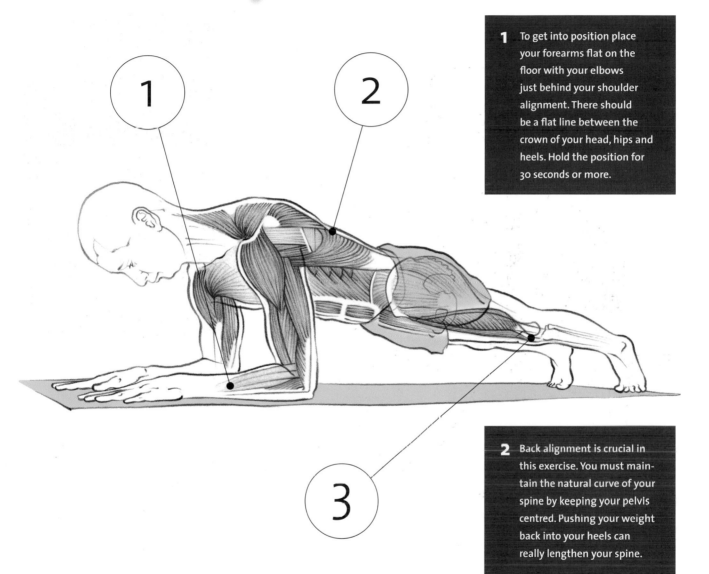

1 To get into position place your forearms flat on the floor with your elbows just behind your shoulder alignment. There should be a flat line between the crown of your head, hips and heels. Hold the position for 30 seconds or more.

2 Back alignment is crucial in this exercise. You must maintain the natural curve of your spine by keeping your pelvis centred. Pushing your weight back into your heels can really lengthen your spine.

3 If you cannot maintain the correct alignment, gently lower your knees to the floor. You should do this for a lower intensity option.

Muscles Used	How will it improve my swimming?
Primary: deep and superficial abs and lower back.	Used by many swimmers in their warm-up routine. You are not working one specific group of muscles but many of the ones you are going to use in the race at the same time.

Core – side plank

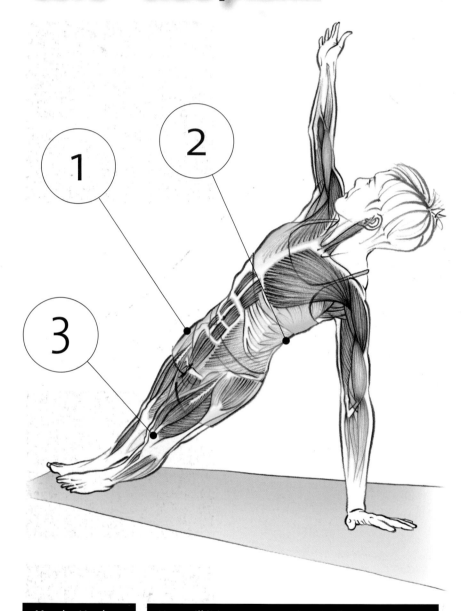

1. To get into position place one hand on the floor with your elbow in a direct line under your shoulder. Your hips should be stacked one on top of the other. Then lift up as if you a drawing away from a flame until your body is in position as per the illustration. Hold for 30 seconds or more.

2. As with the front plank the key is body alignment. Your back must maintain its natural curve – lengthen your legs as the will help to keep your back long.

3. A lower intensity alternative of this exercise is to bend your knees at a right angle so your feet are behind and lift up on your arm while balancing on your knees. This can be used if your shoulders are weak.

Muscles Used	How will it improve my swimming?
Primary: side abs, deep and superficial abs and lower back.	This exercise works on your arms and maintains core strength, which is important in preventing back injuries. Ensure you do it left and right-handed to keep your muscles balanced!

Core – sit-ups

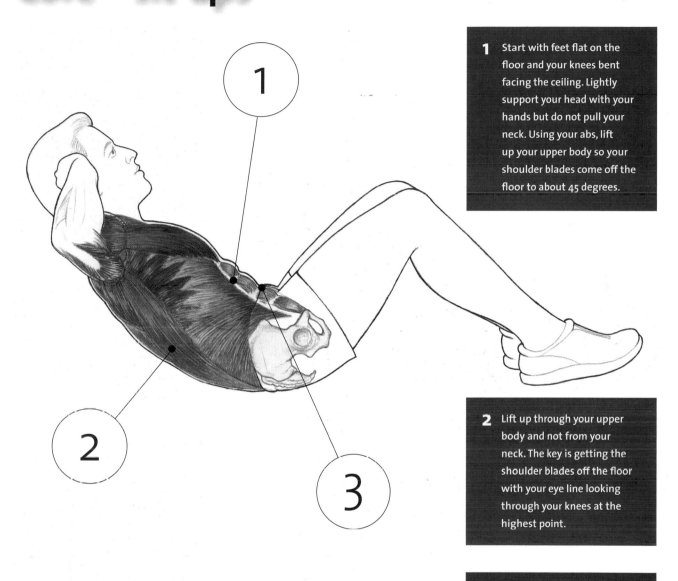

1 Start with feet flat on the floor and your knees bent facing the ceiling. Lightly support your head with your hands but do not pull your neck. Using your abs, lift up your upper body so your shoulder blades come off the floor to about 45 degrees.

2 Lift up through your upper body and not from your neck. The key is getting the shoulder blades off the floor with your eye line looking through your knees at the highest point.

3 To get the best results keep pulling your belly button gently back towards the spine. For increased intensity and to improve balance, this exercise can be done with the base of your back balanced on an exercise ball.

Muscles Used

Primary:
superficial abs.

How will it improve my swimming?

Used, and cursed, by virtually all sportsmen, sit-ups help build up abdominal muscles that will help keep you high up in the water to ensure you are streamlined and more efficient.

Core – shoulder bridge

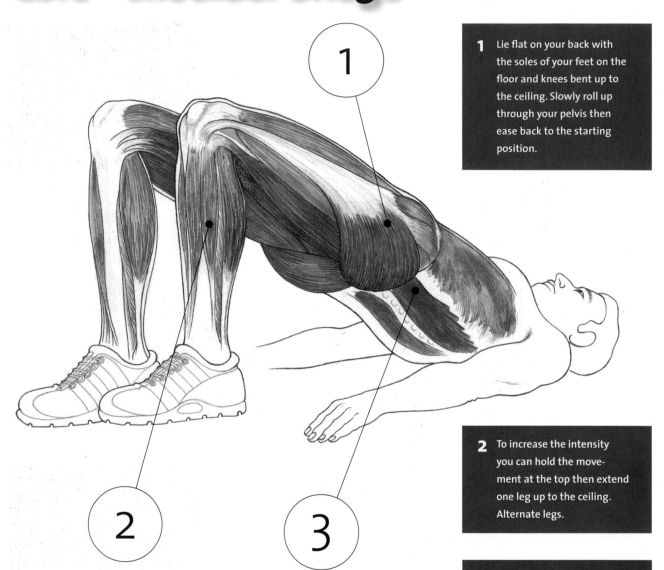

1 Lie flat on your back with the soles of your feet on the floor and knees bent up to the ceiling. Slowly roll up through your pelvis then ease back to the starting position.

2 To increase the intensity you can hold the movement at the top then extend one leg up to the ceiling. Alternate legs.

3 At the top of the movement your shoulders, hips and knees should all be in a line. When rolling up and down, imagine your spine as a bicycle chain and roll through each link one at a time.

Muscles Used	How will it improve my swimming?
Primary: glutes, hamstrings, lower back, abs.	Works your backside and hip muscles that give you the power in your leg kick in all four strokes. You don't actually work your shoulders here but the exercise helps strengthen your back.

Core – leg raises

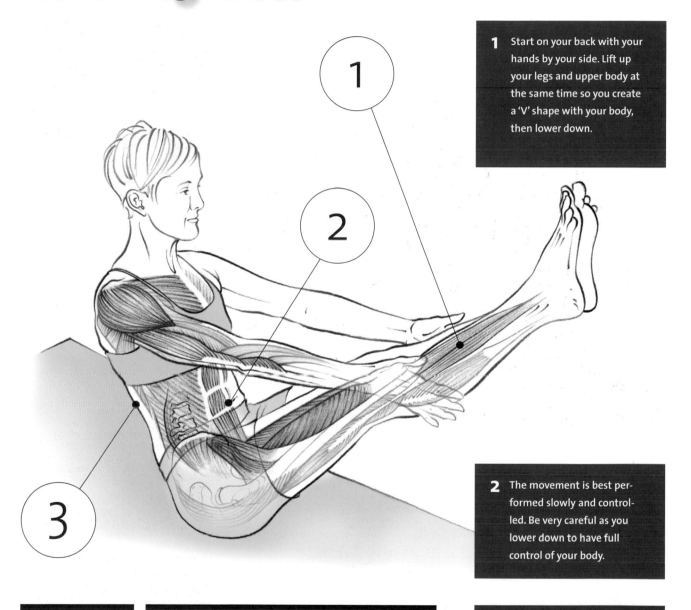

1 Start on your back with your hands by your side. Lift up your legs and upper body at the same time so you create a 'V' shape with your body, then lower down.

2 The movement is best performed slowly and controlled. Be very careful as you lower down to have full control of your body.

3 This is a tough exercise and performed incorrectly can cause injury to the back. A good option to start with is to keep the knees bent as you come up.

Muscles Used	How will it improve my swimming?
Primary: top of leg and abs, hip flexors.	Mainly one for your abdominal muscles, giving similar benefits to sit-ups and maintaining core body strength. Helps develop leg strength and suppleness in your lower back, which is crucial when performing butterfly.

Core – back raises

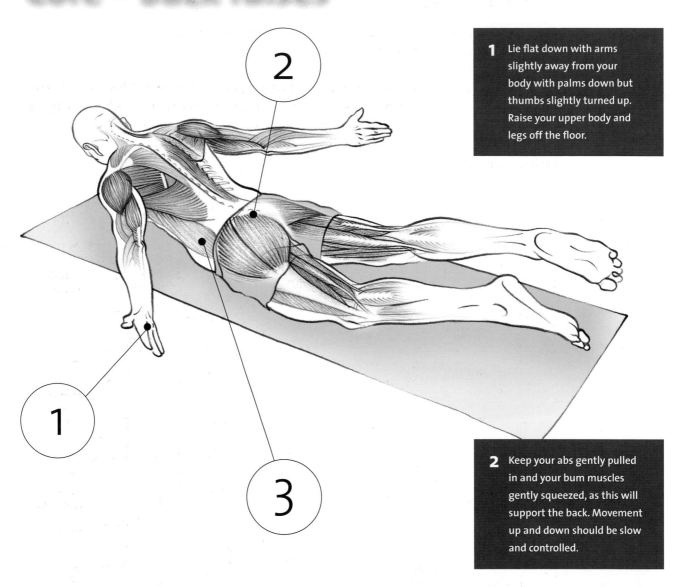

1 Lie flat down with arms slightly away from your body with palms down but thumbs slightly turned up. Raise your upper body and legs off the floor.

2 Keep your abs gently pulled in and your bum muscles gently squeezed, as this will support the back. Movement up and down should be slow and controlled.

3 If you want more support for your back place your hands under your shoulders for support and push up from the floor. Use as much or as little pressure on the hands as you need.

Muscles Used	How will it improve my swimming?
Primary: lower back.	Mimics the up stroke in butterfly and works the muscles in the back, shoulders and legs that generate most of the power in the stroke. Also used in the warm-up by many swimmers.

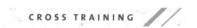

Workout programme – beginners

Sets x2, reps x8-12 (sit-ups, core raises, back raises x15 reps), 1 min recovery between exercises.
Planks: aim for 30 second holds (reduce if losing technique).

To find your ideal weight for each exercise you should be able to complete the reps but just about hit failure on the final rep. As a guide, the heaviest weight you would use would be for your larger muscle groups (eg glutes and quads used in squats) and the lightest weight you would use would be for your smaller muscle groups (eg biceps in bicep curls).

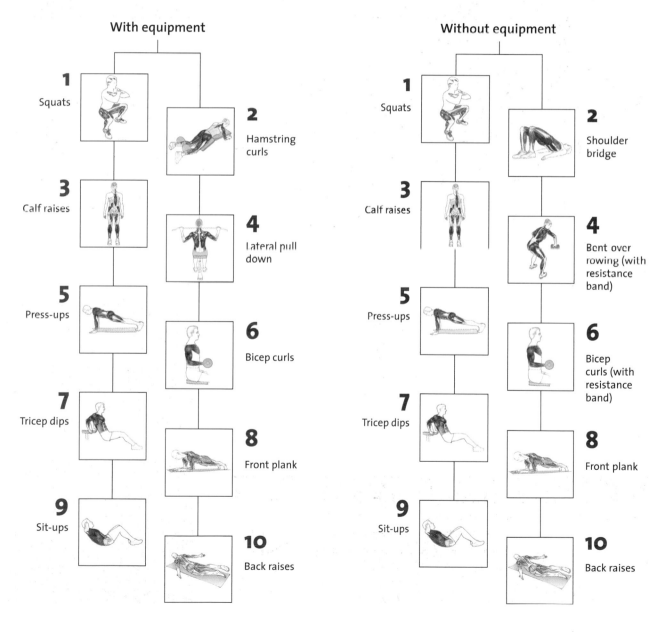

With equipment

1 Squats
2 Hamstring curls
3 Calf raises
4 Lateral pull down
5 Press-ups
6 Bicep curls
7 Tricep dips
8 Front plank
9 Sit-ups
10 Back raises

Without equipment

1 Squats
2 Shoulder bridge
3 Calf raises
4 Bent over rowing (with resistance band)
5 Press-ups
6 Bicep curls (with resistance band)
7 Tricep dips
8 Front plank
9 Sit-ups
10 Back raises

Workout programme – intermediate

Sets x2, reps x10-15 (core raises x20 reps).
Planks: aim for 45 second holds (reduce if losing technique).

To find your ideal weight for each exercise you should be able to complete the reps but just about hit failure on the final rep. As a guide the heaviest weight you would use would be for your larger muscle groups (eg glutes and quads used in squats) and the lightest weight you would use would be for your smaller muscle groups (eg shoulders in dumb-bell raises).

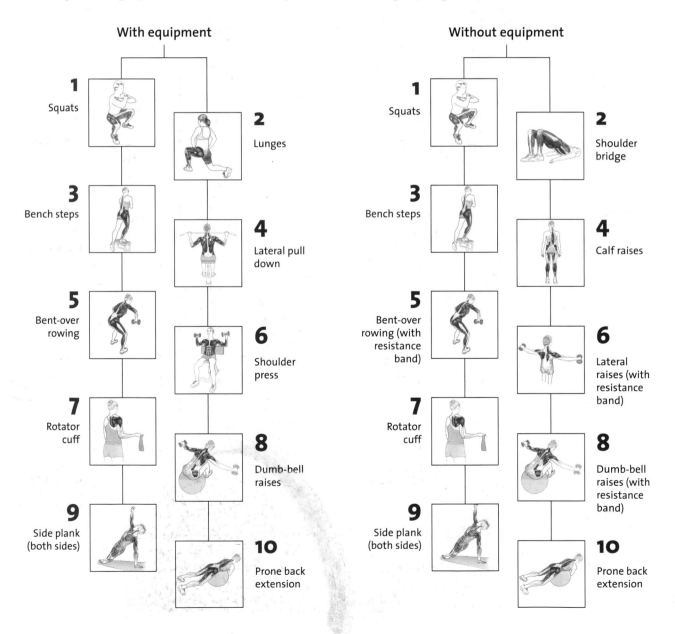

With equipment

1 Squats
2 Lunges
3 Bench steps
4 Lateral pull down
5 Bent-over rowing
6 Shoulder press
7 Rotator cuff
8 Dumb-bell raises
9 Side plank (both sides)
10 Prone back extension

Without equipment

1 Squats
2 Shoulder bridge
3 Bench steps
4 Calf raises
5 Bent-over rowing (with resistance band)
6 Lateral raises (with resistance band)
7 Rotator cuff
8 Dumb-bell raises (with resistance band)
9 Side plank (both sides)
10 Prone back extension

Workout programme – advanced

Sets x3, reps x12-15 (core raises x30 reps).
Planks: aim for 1 min to 1 min and 30 seconds holds (reduce if losing technique).

To find your ideal weight for each exercise you should be able to complete the reps but just about hit failure on the final rep. As a guide, the heaviest weight you would use would be for your larger muscle groups (eg glutes and quads used in squats) and the lightest weight you would use would be for your smaller muscle groups (eg shoulders in dumb-bell raises).

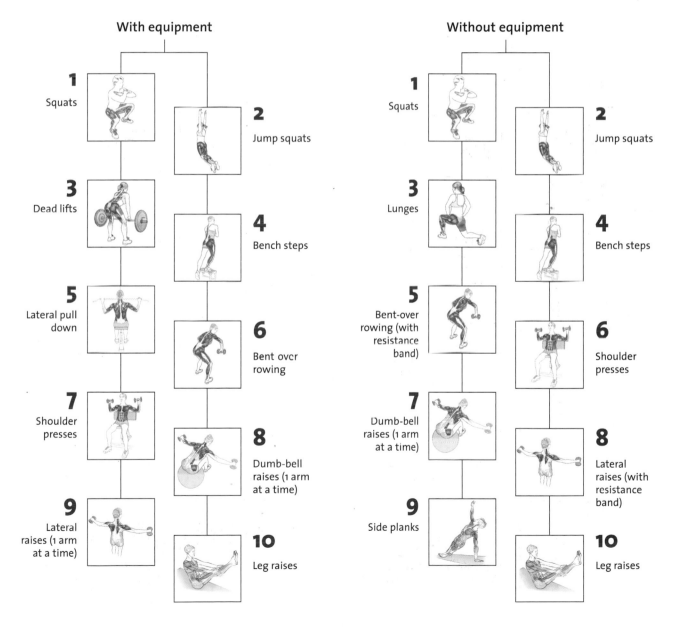

With equipment

1 Squats
2 Jump squats
3 Dead lifts
4 Bench steps
5 Lateral pull down
6 Bent over rowing
7 Shoulder presses
8 Dumb-bell raises (1 arm at a time)
9 Lateral raises (1 arm at a time)
10 Leg raises

Without equipment

1 Squats
2 Jump squats
3 Lunges
4 Bench steps
5 Bent-over rowing (with resistance band)
6 Shoulder presses
7 Dumb-bell raises (1 arm at a time)
8 Lateral raises (with resistance band)
9 Side planks
10 Leg raises

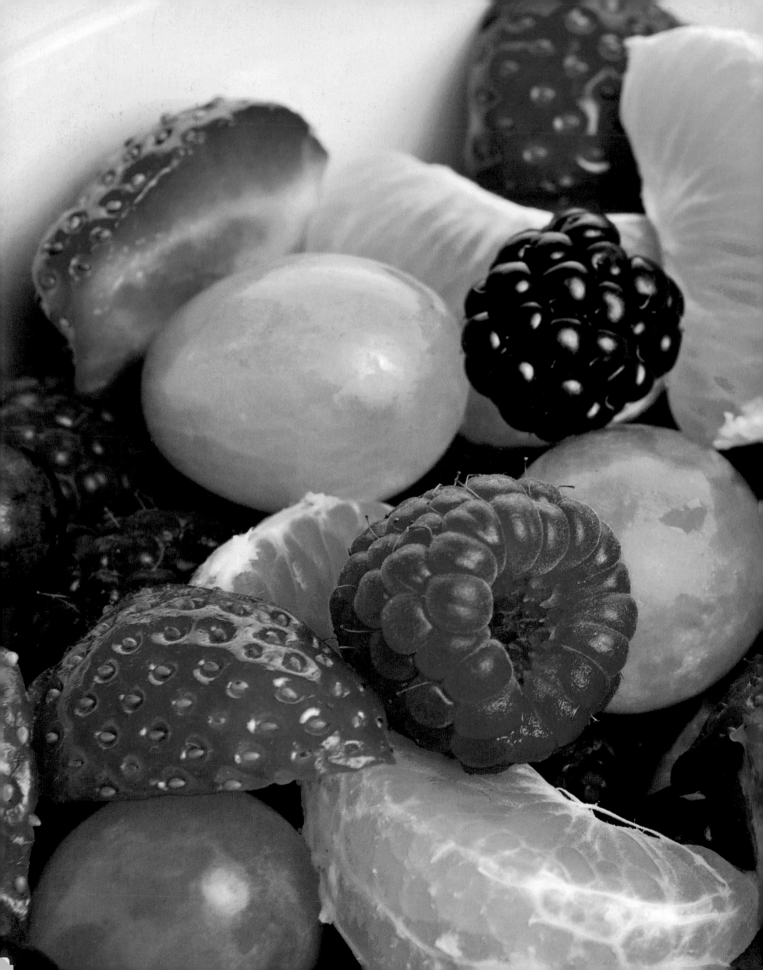

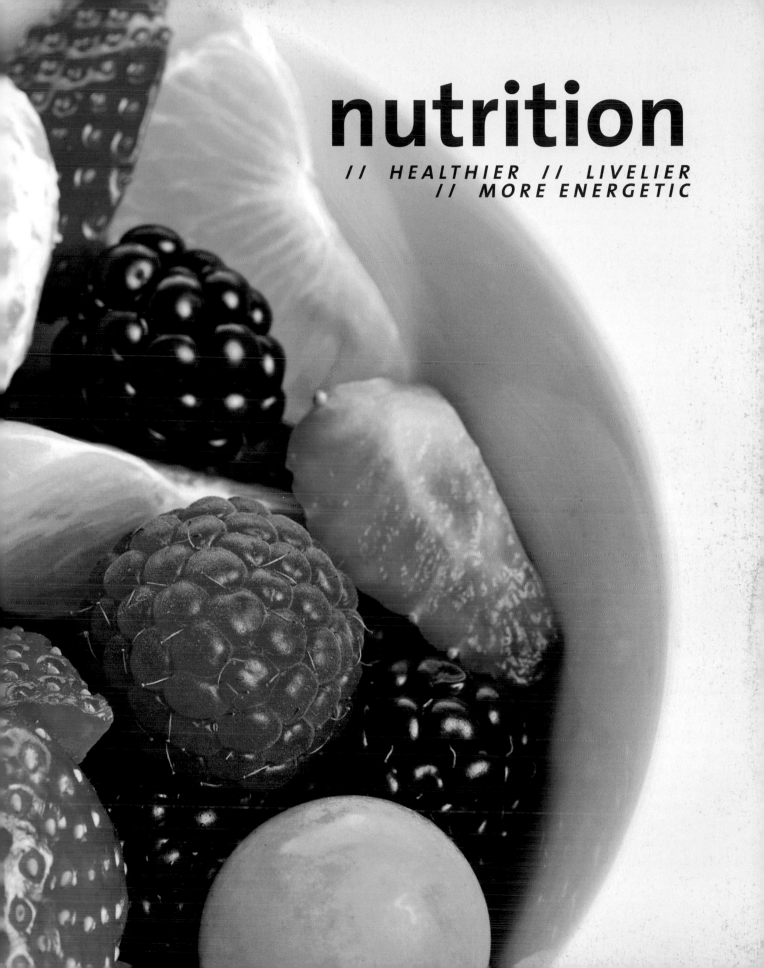

nutrition

// HEALTHIER // LIVELIER // MORE ENERGETIC

The basics

Food and nutrition are the basic elements for a correct training regime in any sport. Think of your body as if it were a car – it could have the most powerful engine, the most aerodynamic shape or the best design but it would never run without its fuel. Food is the natural fuel for your body.

Food can be divided into four basic groups: **carbohydrates, proteins, fats** and **liquids** and each one of them is equally important in running our body, giving it energy, stamina, resistance and self-recovery. Each one of these elements is essential to our nutrition and is absolutely harmless to our health and body if taken in the right amounts, balanced in combination with all the others.

Carbohydrates are the fuel for your muscles. They provide the energy for your muscles to work.

Proteins build and repair muscles whenever they have been stressed during exercise.

Fats are energy stores for your body and help the correct functioning of the cells and maintain your body's temperature.

Liquids maintain the right body fluid concentration and expel toxins.

A correct combination of each one of the above-mentioned elements, adjusted depending on the sport and your body's response, will provide you with the correct nutrition needed, both for training and competition.

A basic diet for an athlete or an active person (someone who trains three times a week for more that 60 minutes per training session) should amount to a daily intake of 3,000–4,500 calories per day, according to the sport and the amount of training. This might seem a lot more than what you heard in your sports club or while chatting when jogging but remember that this diet is not planned in order to make you lose weight but to give you an understanding of what your body needs to perform at its best while under the athletic stress.

If you eat the right foods at the right time, plan your weekly diet with the same care you use to plan your training, weight will never be a problem and you will understand how a correct diet (as a plan to correctly feed your body, instead of a rush into weight loss) will drastically improve your life as well as your athletic performance

Nutrition in sports is as important as the exercise. Again, your body,

as a car, needs the right fuel to perform at its best.

There are four key steps you need to understand before planning your diet:

1. Do not get too hungry as it will make you take the wrong dietary choices and swallow whatever you can find. Have at least five meals a day, calibrating the amounts at each meal.
2. Eat at least three different kinds of foods at each meal as mono-eating will make your body incapable of digesting correctly what you don't usually eat. Choosing different kinds of vegetables, fish and meat, will provide your body with different vitamins and minerals.
3. Always balance the food elements at each meal. Every meal should be based on carbohydrates combined with proteins and fats (amounts change from person to person; but a good starting base is a balance of 50 per cent carbohydrates, 30 per cent proteins and 20 per cent fats).
4. Try to choose foods in their natural state. A banana is better than an energy bar and an orange is better than orange juice for instance.

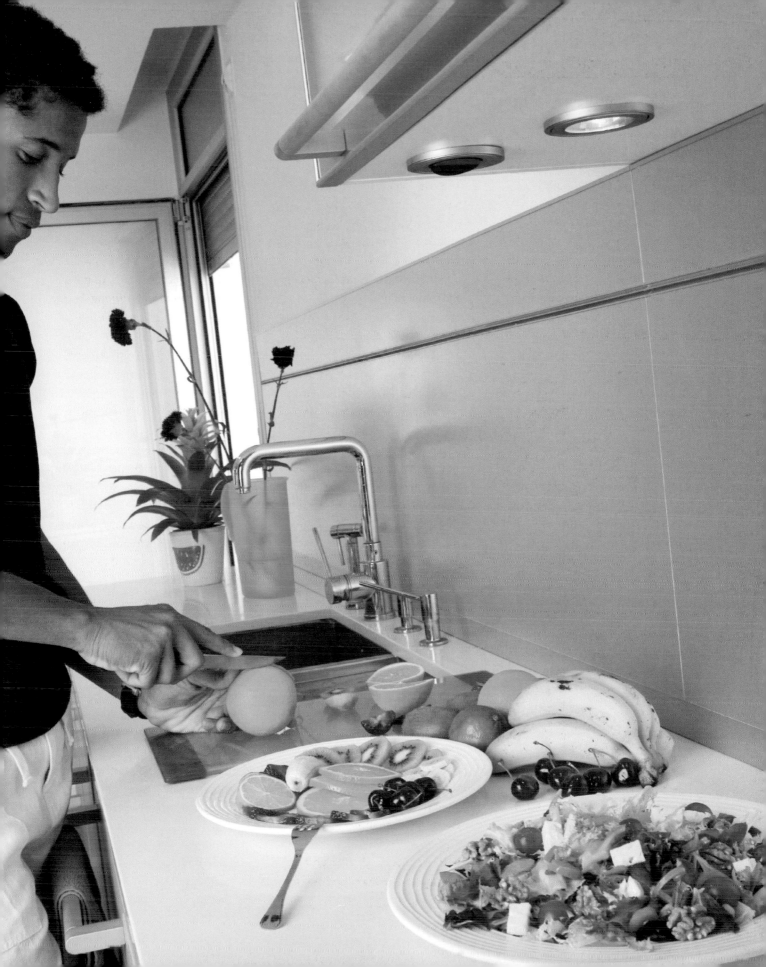

Assess your diet

People tend to be obsessed by their body shape. It is a normal feeling given the kind of images the media world sends us every day. When you assess your ideal diet, try to forget about your shape and think realistically for a moment about what goals you want to achieve athletically. By doing so you will be more focused on understanding, planning and applying the correct diet to everyday life.

First question: do you have breakfast?

Eat breakfast every morning. If you train early in the morning try to wake up half-an-hour before you normally would just to make sure you eat a good amount of food for breakfast. If waking up earlier is going to be impossible, try to eat more carbohydrates the night before, and top up the next morning with some snack. It's very important for you to eat something one hour before training, as it will guarantee the sugars flow in your blood, while the muscles will use the energy stored during the night.

Avoid hyper-protein breakfasts. Remember that every meal should be based around carbohydrates. A little sample of ideal food for breakfast would be:

- Porridge with cottage cheese or ricotta cheese and some nuts.
- A cup of milk or yoghurt over a bowl of cereals with a banana and some raisins. Remember that all-bran cereals tend to be stressful for the bowels, which is inappropriate for training and competition. Also avoid sugar-coated cereals.
- A sandwich made with two slices of whole-grain bread and 60 grams of smoked salmon (you could add a some light cream cheese) and an orange or a glass of orange juice.
- Muesli with yoghurt and one piece of fruit.

If you feel the need for a boost of caffeine, feel free to drink it, as it would not interfere with your training (although it gives stomach acidity to some people). No person is the same, which means it's up to you to find your right intake by calibrating and testing day after day to find the right proportions and taste to suit you.

Second question: do you snack after training?

Remember that eating and drinking after training is the only way you can start to refuel your empty muscles. You can choose what kind of snack you should have, depending on the amount of energy spent and the length of the interval before your next training session. This is the moment where you really train your muscles to intake and store more and more glycogen.

You have two options: either you go for a low or a high GI snack. GI is the acronym for Glycemic Index which is a measure of the effects of carbohydrates on sugar levels. Carbohydrates can be released into the blood slowly (in that case they have a low GI) or quickly (high GI). Although important for the control of illnesses like diabetes, the control of the GI is something that most athletes don't really worry about. What you must decide is the kind of recovery you want from your diet.

If you have two training sessions in one day, or another training session the morning after, then you might want to consider a high GI recovery, choosing food like corn flakes, white bread, watermelon or baked potatoes. On the other hand, it's been shown that a low or medium GI recovery, because of its slower release of sugars, will be more effective in the long run, using food like fruits, vegetables, whole-grain breads, pasta, milk and yoghurt.

Remember that gulping down gallons of protein shakes after training will be almost useless.

You need mainly carbohydrates to refuel your muscles and only some proteins to recover the stressed muscles and help new ones to grow.

Third question: do you ever go hungry during the day?

If you do sometimes go hungry in the day you need adjust your plans to make sure this doesn't happen. Make sure you plan your meals and snacks beforehand by experimenting with your meals for a few days and organize your day around the food you know you will need.

Ideally you should have one substantial breakfast before leaving your house, one snack no longer than four hours after breakfast (between 10.00 and 11.00 for most people), one lunch (if you think it would be better then prepare it the night before, in order to avoid rushing into eating any food you find in the shops when hungry). The have another snack three to four hours later, a good dinner (try to avoid pasta, rice and bread for dinner, unless preparing for a competition or the night before the competition itself) and one last evening snack.

Fourth question: do you find yourself fatigued during training?

There could be different reasons for being fatigued during training.

- A low glycogen storage. The glycogen has been burned and you are now using your proteins and fats as fuel, provoking your blood to carry ketones to your brain. In this case you should eat more carbohydrates before training and more carbohydrates after training, in order to teach your muscles to store as much glycogen as possible.
- Dehydration. A lack of liquids means your body can't cool down properly, endangering the health of you cells and making the expulsion of carbon dioxide and lactic acid more difficult.

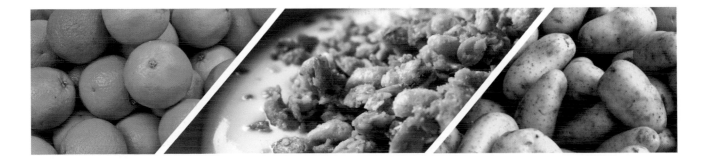

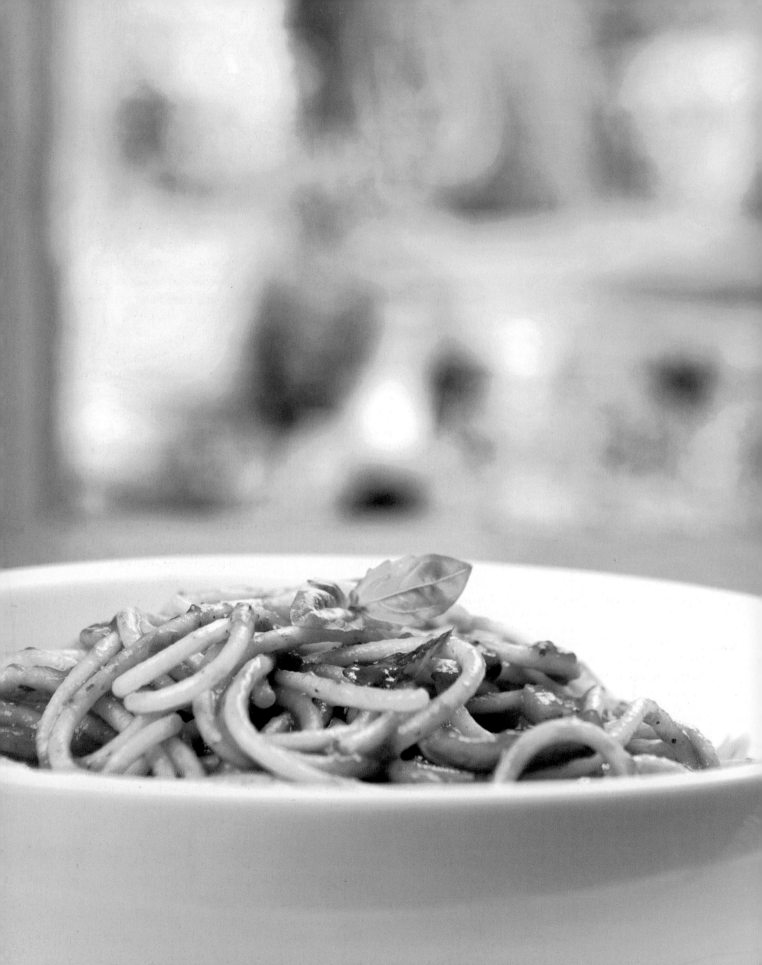

Carbohydrates

One of the many myths you may have read is that carbohydrates are fattening. This is untrue. Fats are fattening, carbohydrates are the basic fuel you need to eat in order to have enough energy in your muscles. In a sports diet carbohydrates are an absolute must of your nutrition requirements.

Carbohydrates can be divided into two groups: simple and complex. Simple carbohydrates are monosaccharides (single-sugar molecules: fructose, glucose and galactose) and disaccharides (double-sugar molecules: table sugar, milk sugar, honey and refined syrups). Fruits and vegetables contain many different kinds of carbohydrates, which is one of the reasons why your diet should include a good variety of vegetables and fruits.

During digestion your stomach turns the sugars and carbohydrates into glucose, before the latter is then turned into a polymer (a chain of five or more sugar molecules) called glycogen. Glycogen is the key to your energy levels. Glycogen gets stored in your muscles and your liver, supplying your body with the right amount of energy for your training or your competition.

While the glycogen stored in your muscles will function as an energy reserve to move your body and train your muscles, the one stored in your liver will provide a slow-release of sugars into your bloodstream, guaranteeing a constant amount of sugars to your brain. This is important, because the sugars in your brain will influence your performance drastically.

Did you ever hear about, or ever hit the infamous 'wall'? The wall is something many professional athletes have hit during their career. It's a moment during which you become sure you are not going to make it to the finish. The wall is not a metaphysical concept, it is simply the moment when you have no more sugars flowing to your brain. Having the right amount of glycogen stored in both your muscles and your liver will help you avoid the wall.

What is the main difference between the different sugars, then? While refined sugars, soft drinks and energy drinks will only provide an energy supply, vegetables and fruits will supply, along with different amounts of glucose, also vitamins and minerals which will help spark and run your body engine in the correct way.

Always try to eat foods in their natural state. Whole-wheat breads, brown rice, brown pasta, as all the nutritional elements you will find in unrefined products, are more valuable than the ones you will find in refined ones. The same concept can be applied to cooked carbohydrates – it is preferable to undercook vegetables, in order for them to retain the vitamins and minerals contained in them along with the sugars and starches. This leads to a very important point you should be aware of. Your muscles need to be trained not only through exercise, but also by making them capable of storing the biggest amount of glycogen possible. How do you do that? By eating the right carbohydrates in the right amount.

During training you put your muscles under stress in order to grow them and make them stronger. At the same time, by supplying them with the right amount of carbohydrates, you will teach them to store more glycogen.

In 100 grams of untrained muscle you can store only 13 grams of glycogen but the same amount of trained muscle will store about 32 grams, while a muscle trained to be loaded with carbohydrates will be able to store between 35 and 40 grams. Needless to say, the latter is the muscle that will perform better and for longer.

Carbohydrates

1 Unrefined food will have a better nutritional value than the refined ones. Wild rice, whole-wheat breads, brown pasta, popcorn (unbuttered), oats and porridge, raw fruits and vegetables, etc.

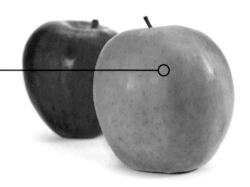

2 Always make sure that any meal you take during the day is based around carbohydrates. Try to think in terms of the proportions stated above (50-30-20).

3 Vary your food as much as possible. A good way is to plan your meals by colour (green leaves or broccoli, tomatoes, peppers, carrots, oranges, apples, blueberries, etc).

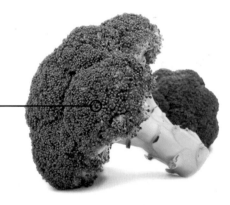

4 Always make sure that before and after training you have the right amount of carbohydrates to restore your energy levels and sugars in your bloodstream. Once the glycogen is used up your body will start burning your fat as an energy supplement. Although this is the basic concept of how to trim down your stomach, bear in mind that such a process is detrimental to your performance, as your bloodstream will carry ketons to your brain instead of sugars, amplifying your tiredness and affecting your mood.

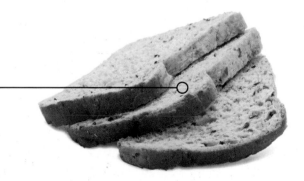

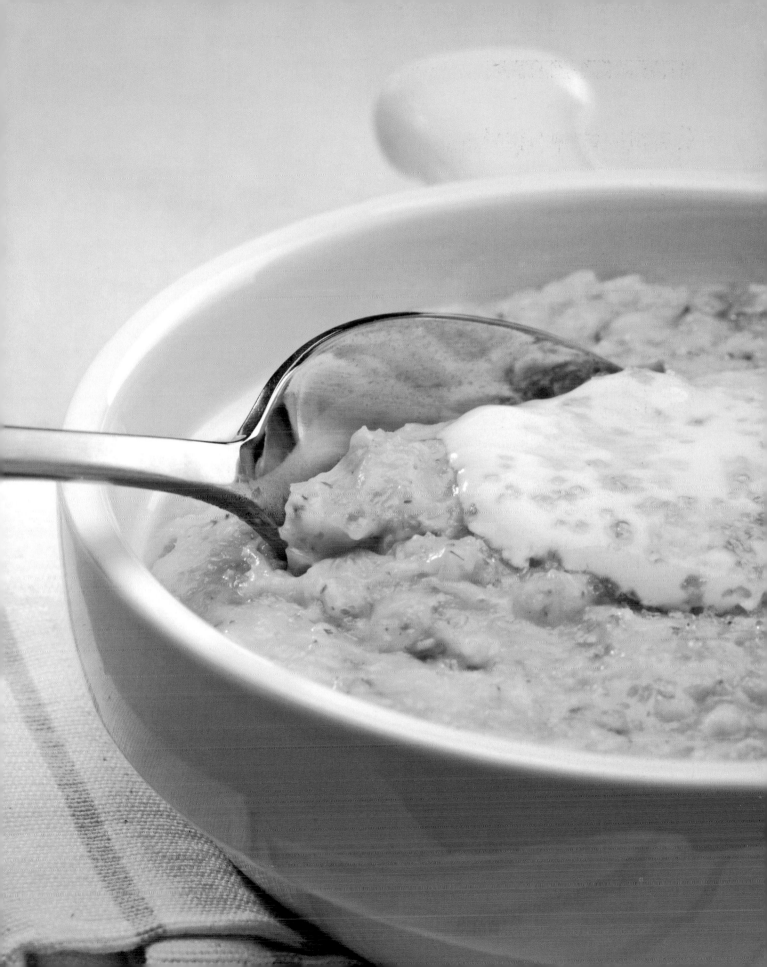

Proteins

Let's start by refuting another myth: proteins do not make you stronger, exercise does. There is always a magic aura around words such as proteins and amino acids, believed to be the mysterious ingredients to a muscular body. Don't worry, it's not so mysterious.

Proteins have many different roles in your body. They help build new muscles, repair those stressed by exercise, are the reason your hair and nails grow, energize your immune system and, above all, help replace red blood cells. A protein-based diet is useless. Drinking protein shakes, eating too many egg whites, or stuffing yourself with chicken breast will lead to poor results. An over-intake of proteins can be useless, even counterproductive. Your body can store only a certain amount of protein or amino acids and if you exceed this they will be either burned for energy (a scarce amount if compared to carbohydrates) when the body runs out, or stored as glycogen or fat. There are two main problems you can face if following a diet with too much protein.

1. It will prevent you from eating the right amount of carbohydrates, lowering the amount of energy stored in your muscles.
2. It will break down into urea, an organic compound your body eliminates through urine. People who eat too many proteins will need to increase their fluid intake to eliminate as much urea as possible, leading to frequent visits to the toilet.

By eating too many proteins you also increase the chance of eating excessive fats (through meats, and condiments) that your body will store. The correct amount of protein an athlete can digest varies but as a rule of thumb, is calculated to be between 1.2 and 1.6 grams per body weight kilogram per day. That is usually less than your daily intake by only eating meat, fish, dairy products or legumes. The ideal intake would be a daily total of about 150g to 200g, adding the proteins you should get from two servings of low-fat dairy products (milk, yoghurt and cheese) per day.

Meats can be divided in three kinds: white meats, red meats and fish. An ideal sports diet should include all kinds of meats in your weekly plan.
- Fish is the best option as the fats it contains are unsaturated (including the famous Omega-3), so is a better choice than the saturated fats commonly found in meats and dairy products.
- White meat is preferable to red meat as it usually contains less fat (if it is either breast or properly skinned thigh and drumsticks).
- Lean red meat, although not the healthiest option, should be eaten between three and four times per week. Red meat contains iron and zinc and iron is an essential part of haemoglobin, a protein that transports oxygen to your muscles and brain. If you are missing the right amount of iron you could suffer fatigue and exhaustion. Zinc is a mineral that plays a big role in removing carbon dioxide from your muscles when you are exercising. A good red meat is venison as it contains a lower quantity of saturated fat.

With dairy products you should eat low-fat. Semi-skimmed milk and yoghurt are close to the ideal intake percentage (they contain a percentage of 40 per cent carbohydrates, 35 per cent proteins, 25 per cent fats), so are a perfect snack. It's an easy way to eat proteins and also supply vitamin D and calcium and the right amount of potassium, phosphorus and riboflavin. Potassium and phosphorus help your body in metabolizing the calcium to strengthen your bones, while riboflavin is a vitamin that helps your body to transform the food into energy.

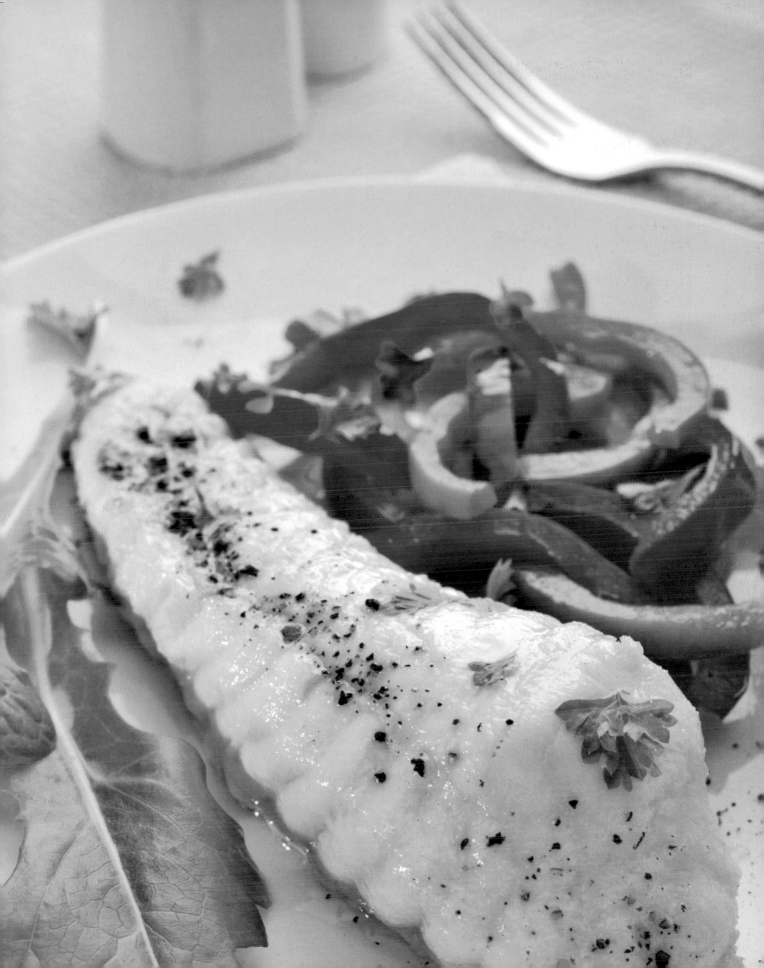

Proteins

1 Choose fish before white meat or red meat, but make sure you eat all three kinds during the week.

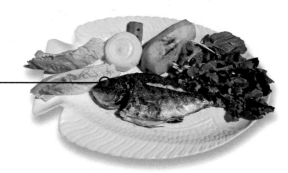

2 Include proteins in every meal.

3 You can find all the proteins you need in the food you eat – you don't need to use shakes, bars or pills.

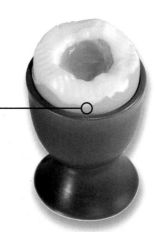

4 Try to eat low-fat dairy products at least once, preferably twice a day.

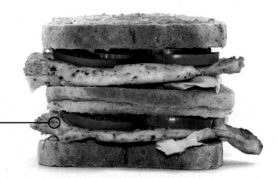

5 Do not overfeed yourself with proteins, as it is pointless.

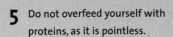

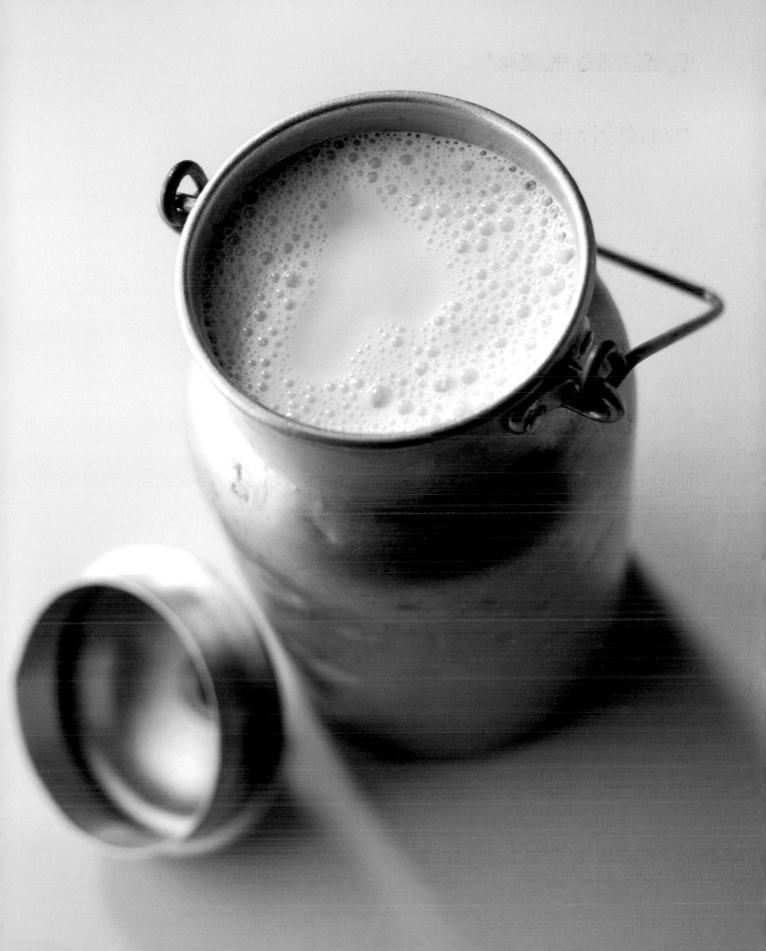

Fats

Fat is as important in your diet as any other food element. Fat helps provide the temperature regulation of your body, helps the health of skin and hair and provides a safety coating for your internal organs.

The most important thing is to know what kinds of fat you should eat and in what quantities. Fats can be divided into hard fats and soft fats. Hard fats are the fats that come in the form of meat lard, chicken skin or butter, while soft fats, the ones you should favour in your diet, are in the form of olive oil and canola oil.

As mentioned earlier, calories from fat should correspond to about 20 per cent of your diet. The most important thing to remember is to stay away from Hydrogenated Trans

Fats, which are a very unhealthy result of a chemical process that adds hydrogen to both mono and polyunsaturated fats.

Don't be afraid of eating fats during your resting periods. Many people think if you don't exercise your muscles will turn into fat and you will gain weight. That is untrue. Muscles and fat are two distinct components of your body and you will only gain weight by taking more calories from fat than the ones you are burning, which, in the doses that have been mentioned before, is very unlikely.

You might have seen people in the gym torturing their abs, hoping to lose their belly by over-exercising the part closest to it. What you need to understand is that you lose

your excessive fat by exercising the whole body and consuming the calories that you have taken. Let's put it this way: if you want to lose fat, you need to grow your muscles (in the whole body), as bigger muscles consume more calories. Don't try to over-stress specific areas of your body, as this is useless.

Remember that fats are what gives taste to your food, helping to make it more favourable to your palate. As you are making an effort to stick to a dietary plan for your athletic training, try to enjoy it as much as possible, adding the right amount of healthy fats to your meals.

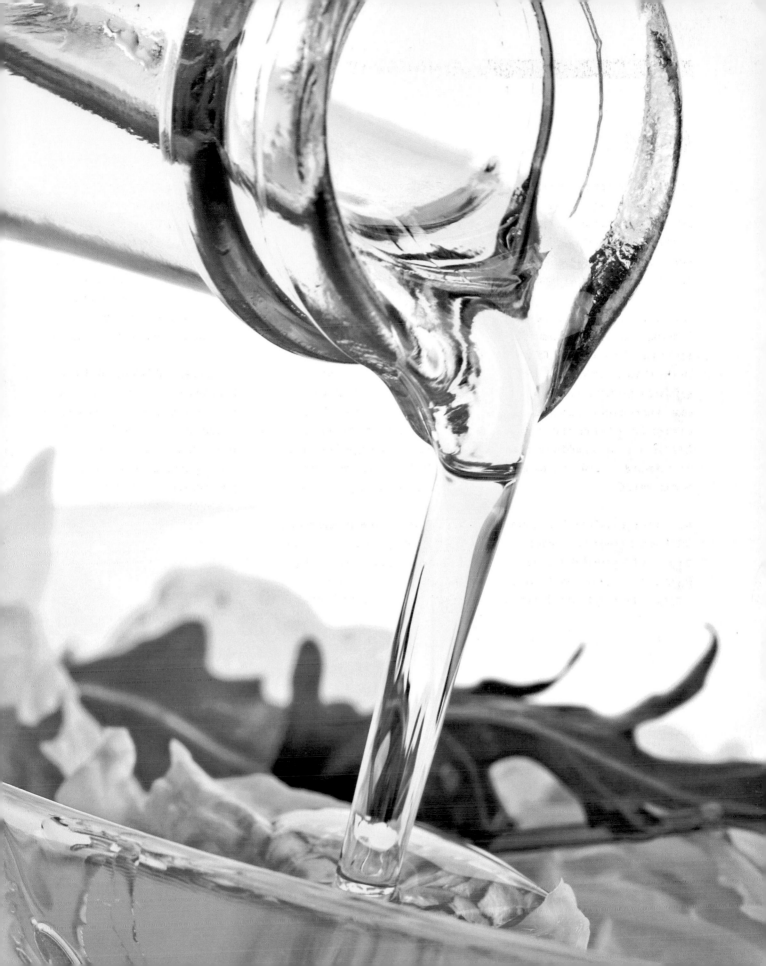

Fats

1 Olive oil is a monounsaturated fat and is the best choice. Always try to buy extra-virgin olive oil and use it to cook and dress any food you want. The ideal amount should be around two teaspoons for each meal.

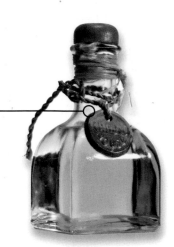

2 Nuts – like walnuts, almonds, pistachios, macadamia, Brazilian nuts, pine kernels, olives – are also a good choice for fat intake. Each one of them is a different size and contains a different amount of fat, so it's important to weigh them so you know approximately how many you need. For example: cashew nuts, peanuts, almonds, pine kernels, require a dose of nine grams per meal while walnuts, macadamias, hazelnuts, pecans and pistachios are about seven to eight grams per meal. For avocado and green olives allow a bit more (about 18 grams for the avocado and 30 grams for the olives).

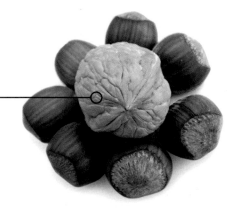

3 Fish oil is another good choice, as it is rich in healthy fats. However, not many people like the taste and it would be a pity to waste a whole meal because of it.

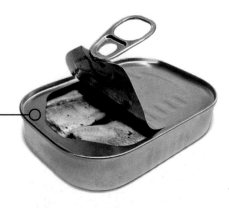

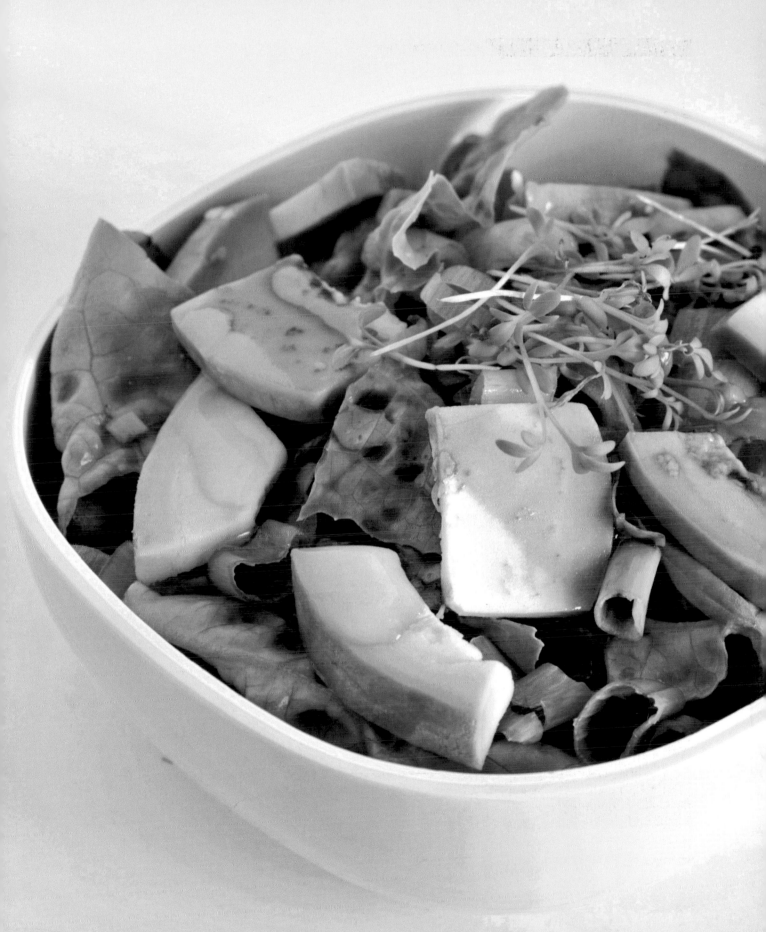

Liquids

Water is the base of life. Your body is made in the most part by liquids and any loss of liquids has to be quickly restored.

Water does the following.
- It keeps your blood liquid, helping the correct transportation of oxygen, glucose and fat, while taking away carbon dioxide and lactic acid.
- It helps keep your body cool by absorbing heat from your muscles, sweating the heat out, cooling the skin through evaporating sweat and allowing the cooled down epidermis to cool the blood that cools down the organs. It's a positive vicious cycle.

Thirst is the most common sensation our body delivers to make us aware that we need to restore our balance. This sensation becomes more complicated when we deal with sports however.

There are many variables to be taken into consideration when you are exercising. There is the level of preparation, the weather, the fact your mind is focused on a goal, your body is too well trained or, because of the water on your body, you don't feel the heat. Bear in mind that, while exercising, your brain will communicate 'thirst' to you when you have already lost about

one per cent of liquids and then it might be too late to rehydrate yourself. At that point your heart is beating more than needed, burning more glycogen than it should. At a two per cent loss you are officially dehydrated and at three per cent your body could be impaired in continuing the task.

The secret is to plan your drinking as well as your eating. Evaluate the amount of liquids you lose during a training session. To do so, weigh yourself naked before the training and right after, before drinking. The difference in weight will tell you the amount of liquids you lost. Your urine should always be a pale yellow; if it is dark and dense it means that there are too many metabolic wastes compared to the amount of water.

For swimmers, who can't stop during a race to drink, it is necessary to pre-plan the water intake before getting into the pool. Once you have established the amount of water you sweat during your exercise, you can start introducing extra liquids into your body beforehand, so that at the end of the training session you will need less water to re-establish your correct hydration.

It takes between eight and 12 hours before your body becomes fully rehydrated so always plan your

drinking during both your everyday life and training. By sweating you not only lose liquids but also electrolytes such as magnesium, potassium, sodium and calcium.

Always start you training session fully rehydrated from the session before by drinking between five and eight millilitres per kilo of your body weight. You can add sodium to your drink or chose a sodium enhanced drink, as it might help retain the water in your body.

You can use sodium in food and beverages after your training if you need to rehydrate quickly for a second session (up to 12 hours after the first one). Drinking between 30 per cent and 50 per cent more fluids than the ones you lost during exercise should be enough to re-establish the right concentration of liquids in your body.

Try to stay away from alcohol as much as possible. It causes strong dehydration as it is a potent diuretic and it would make you waste more liquids than you should. Also remember alcohol is a depressant and it suppresses drastically your motor skills along with your mood.

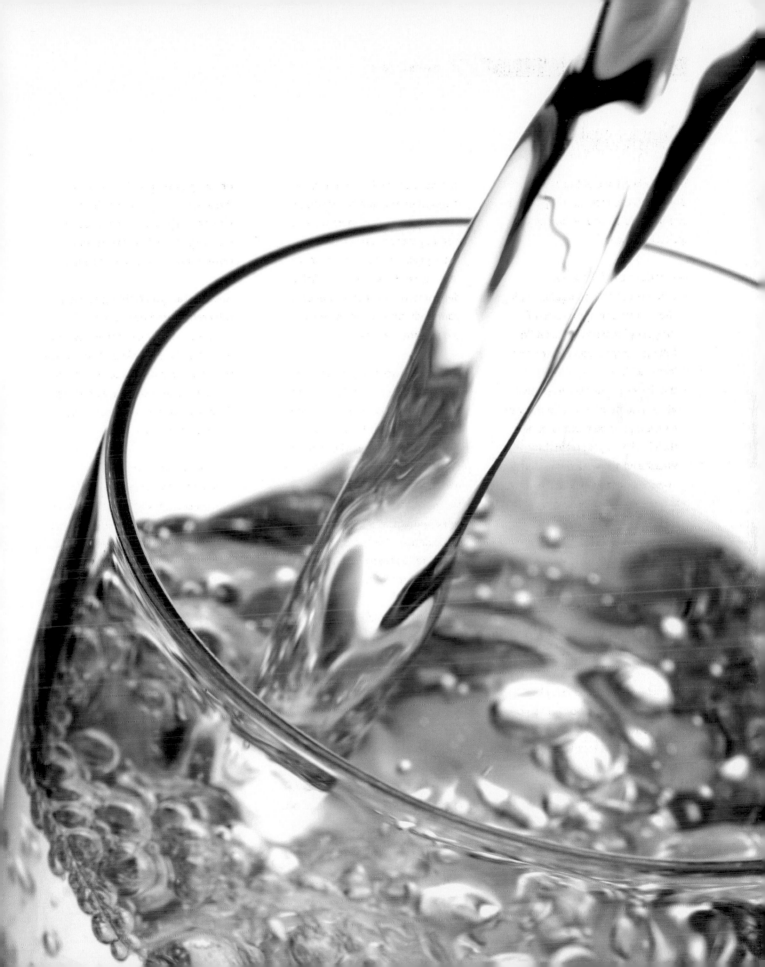

Pre- and post-competition planning

Before the competition

Your pre-competition training should be winding down (tapering) in the few days before the event (see Training programmes page 144). This is because your muscles need time to recover from hard exercise. During this time, while you are reducing your training load you should be re-establishing the glycogen in your muscles, rehydrating yourself and mending the stressed muscles by eating some proteins.

Try to interpret your pre-competition training as a final rehearsal for the real event. Some people think that stuffing themselves with pasta the night before the competition will be enough but things are a bit more complicated than that.

During training you will have taught your muscles to store a good amount of glycogen in order to have a good reserve in every training session. The more you train your muscles with exercise, the more glycogen your muscles will be able to store, if educated to receive it.

From one or two weeks before your competition you should slowly increase the amount of carbohydrates by about 100 grams per day. The day before the competition

itself you should start loading your body with carbohydrates from breakfast time.

Every athlete reacts differently to a competition. Some have no problem having a good dinner the night before – others find it difficult to digest because of the excitement or worry. Therefore, start loading yourself with carbohydrates from breakfast. And, if you feel like eating dinner try to vary the type of carbohydrates as much as you can. Pasta by itself might do the trick, but remember that fruits and vegetables contain slow sugar-releasing carbohydrates and they will help for endurance the day after. Avoid bran flakes or anything that you know could lead to stomach problems.

Swimming has, for nutrition, an upside and a downside. The upside is that it's a sport that doesn't affect your stomach and bowels like jogging or football, as the movement of the body is smooth and not jumpy. The downside is that during a race it is impossible to stop to refill your muscles and re-balance your liquids.

On the morning of the competition, according to the time the event starts, there are few rules you need to follow.

- Make sure you wake up in the morning with the right fluid balance. You can easily determine it by the colour of your urine.

- Start by having a big glass of water and breakfast or, if the competition is too early to have breakfast, make sure you load some more carbohydrates one hour before the event. This will make sure that your liver will produce enough sugar to be delivered to your brain throughout the duration of the competition.

- Drink your water between one to two hours before the race so you can expel it before the race starts.

After the competition

As you will have seen, after the event you need to let your body recover by rebalancing the glycogen and the fluids. In swimming it is tricky to determine the amount of fluids you lost through sweat, so be sure you weigh yourself before and after the competition. Take advantage of the first hour after the event, as it will be the period when you body will assimilate all the nutrients best.

Carbohydrates mixed with a little protein is the best option to have both glycogen delivered to

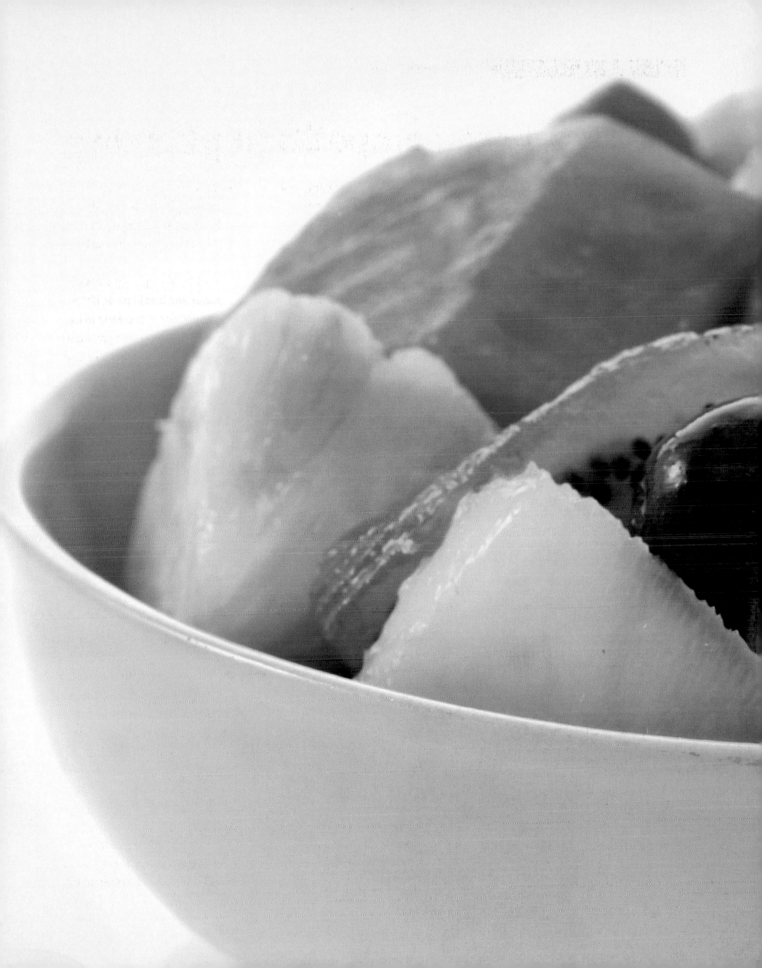

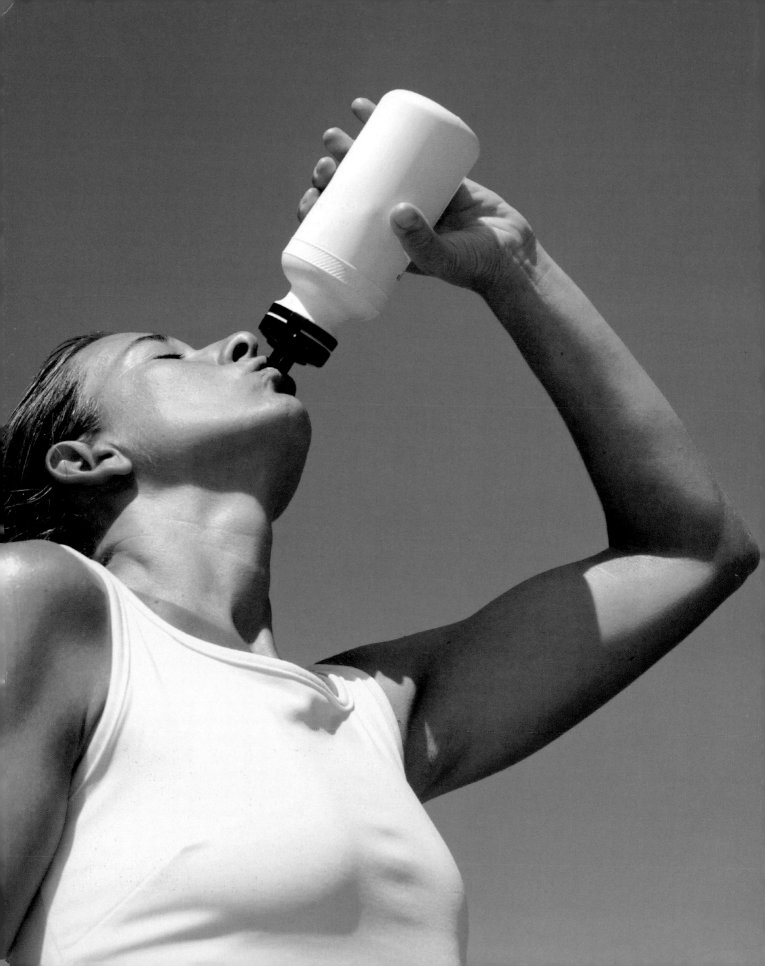

your muscles while reducing the emission of cortisol, the hormone that breaks down your muscles during exercise.

According to whether you will have a short or a long time before the next competition, you will have to find the right way to fully recover your muscles and blood. Swimming often faces you with the problem of back-to-back events and recovering has to be planned carefully.

Different athletes prefer different solutions according to their experience. The main thing is to plan a good nutrition schedule. If you know you will have to face three competitions in 40 hours, you might want to plan your diet starting from the week before, in such way that it will be faster to recover between the events.

If you have two events back to back you want to make sure you will recover immediately after the first one by over-loading yourself with high-GI carbohydrates and liquids that will restore not only the fluids but also the electrolytes (some sport drinks do that). Try to drink as much as possible and judge the level of rehydration from the colour of your urine and comparing your weight before and after the event. If you happen to have more than two competitions in a span of more than two days, keep in mind that low-GI carbohydrates have been proven to be more effective in the long run.

If you have enough time to recover after the event (one week), make sure you rebalance your fluids and have a little snack combining carbo-hydrates and proteins in the usual balance and then take your time, by simply starting the nutritional plan where you left it before the prepa-ration to the competition.

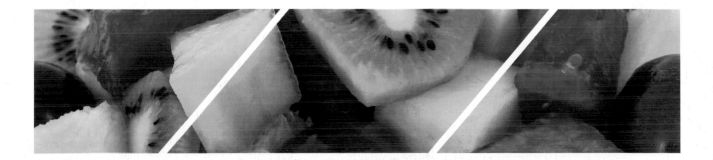

Recipes

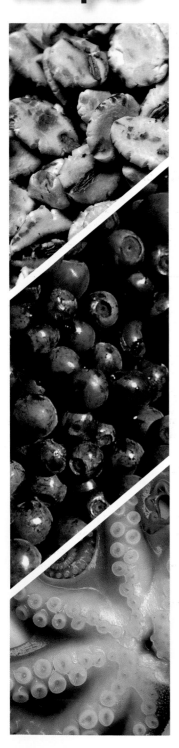

OATS, RICOTTA AND PISTACHIOS

Ingredients
- *50 grams rolled oats*
- *140 grams of ricotta cheese*
- *8-10 pistachios, no shells*
- *Pinch of salt or honey*

Preparation Boil the oats in water until reaching your preferred consistency. In a bowl, mix the cooked oats, the ricotta cheese and pistachios. Add either a pinch of salt or half teaspoon of honey, depending on whether you prefer savoury or sweet. This is a perfect balanced snack, which combines proteins, carbohydrates and fat.

COTTAGE CHEESE WITH WARM BLUBERRY AND WALNUTS

Ingredients
- *220 grams of blueberries*
- *1 teaspoon of fructose*
- *70 grams of low-fat cottage cheese*
- *3 walnuts*

Preparation Warm the blueberries in a saucepan over low heat with fructose and a little bit of water and keep stirring gently until the berries are softened. Place the cottage cheese in a bowl and pour the fruits over it. Sprinkle with the crumbled walnuts. Perfect as a snack.

STUFFED SQUID

Ingredients
- *1 big squid (200 grams cleaned – keep the tentacles)*
- *2 teaspoons of chopped parsley and a little chopped garlic*
- *250 grams of grated fresh whole-grain bread or whole-grain breadcrumbs*
- *30 grams of grated Parmesan cheese*
- *1 tablespoon of olive oil*

Preparation Keep the squid body intact. For the filling: chop the tentacles and add them to a bowl along with the parsley, garlic, fresh breadcrumbs and Parmesan. Start pounding the mixture with your hands and add water and oil as needed. Fill the squid with the mix and close it with a toothpick. Put it in the oven for 30 minutes, using any leftover paste to coat the squid. Serve with a side of salad or a piece of fruit cut up.

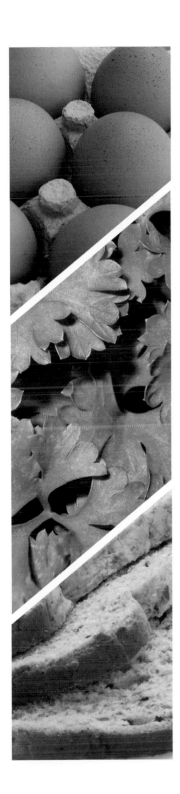

BUTTER-FREE EGGS FLORENTINE

Ingredients
- *300 grams of spinach*
- *White wine vinegar*
- *35 grams of cottage cheese*
- *2 slices of whole-grain bread, toasted*
- *2 eggs, poached*
- *Salt and pepper to taste*
- *Grated Parmesan cheese or shredded mild Cheddar cheese*

Preparation Boil spinach until lightly soft. Mix a teaspoon of vinegar to the cottage cheese and mix well. Place spinach over the two slices of toasted bread. Arrange cooked, drained eggs over the top of the spinach then pour the cottage cheese over the eggs. Sprinkle with salt, pepper and grated Parmesan cheese.

SPICY OATS WITH GRILLED CHICKEN BREAST (OR VENISON STEAK)

Ingredients
- *3 teaspoons olive oil*
- *1/2 red onion*
- *Pinch of chilli powder, pinch of paprika, 1 bay leaf*
- *1 garlic clove*
- *350 grams of raw oats (in grains)*
- *Grilled chicken breast or 120 gram venison steak*
- *Parsley*

Preparation Mix olive oil and 3 tablespoons of water in a cooking pan. Chop up the onion and cook it in the oily water adding chilli powder, paprika, the bay leaf and garlic until golden. Add oats and let them roast a bit. Then add water and let them cook for 30 minutes. While it's cooking grill the chicken breast or venison steak. Serve with a sprinkle of chopped parsley.

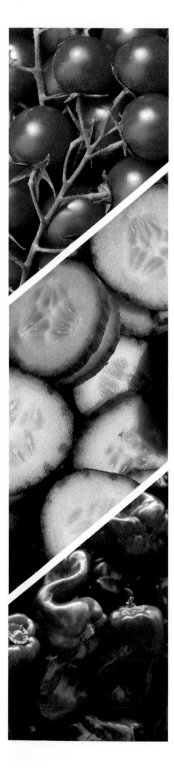

FRESH SALAD

Ingredients
- *300 grams of cherry tomatoes*
- *300 grams of cucumber*
- *1/4 red onion, softened in warm water and a teaspoon of vinegar*
- *300 grams of low-fat Greek yoghurt*
- *2 teaspoons olive oil*
- *Salt and pepper to taste*
- *Pinch chives and dill*
- *Paprika to taste*

Preparation Cut the cherry tomatoes in half and the cucumbers into cubes. Mix the cherry tomatoes, cucumber, onion and Greek yogurt in a salad bowl. Add olive oil, salt and pepper, and sprinkle with chives, dill and paprika according to taste. Perfect and easy to make.

VENISON STEW

Ingredients
- *140 grams diced venison*
- *Salt and black pepper to taste*
- *1 tablespoon chopped fresh thyme*
- *3 tablespoons olive oil*
- *1 chopped onion*
- *300 grams chopped celery*
- *120 grams chopped carrots*
- *1 tablespoon chopped garlic*
- *200 grams chopped tomatoes*
- *150 grams chopped red peppers*
- *2 bay leaves*
- *1 glass red wine*
- *1 slice whole-grain bread, toasted*

Preparation In a mixing bowl, toss the venison with salt and black pepper, half the thyme and a little sprinkle of oil. In a large pot, over a high heat, add the rest of the olive oil. When the oil is hot, sear the meat for 2 to 3 minutes, stirring occasionally. Add the onions and let them cook for 4 minutes. Add the celery and carrots. Season with salt and pepper. Sauté for 4 minutes. Add the garlic, tomatoes, red peppers, the rest of the thyme, and bay leaves to pan. When the water from the vegetables is evaporated add the red wine. Add some boiling water if needed. Bring the liquid up to a boil, cover and reduce to a simmer. Simmer the stew for 45 minutes to 1 hour, or until the meat is very tender. If the liquid evaporates too much add a little more. Serve on a shallow bowl over a slice of whole-grain toasted bread.

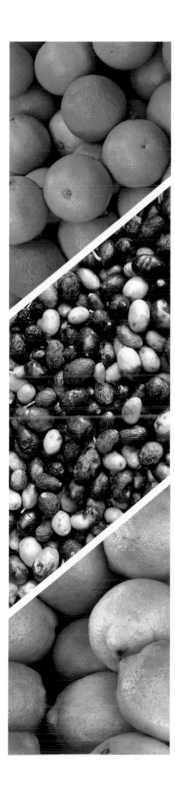

LEMON SOLE WITH FENNEL AND ORANGE SALAD

Ingredients
- *1 pinch sea salt*
- *1 pinch smoked paprika*
- *1 pinch ground cinnamon*
- *Dill*
- *2 teaspoons of olive oil*
- *1 lemon sole (200 grams)*

For the fennel and orange salad
2 bulbs fennel, thinly sliced
1/2 red onion, finely sliced
1 orange, sliced and then cut into quarters
2 teaspoons of olive oil

Preparation Preheat the oven to 190°C (370°F)/gas 5. Mix together sea salt, smoked paprika, cinnamon and dill. Coat the lemon sole in the spice mixture. Lightly grease a cooking foil sheet with a little olive oil and place in a baking tray. Place the sole on the foil and then close the foil, joining the sides together. Let the fish cook for 10-12 minutes according to taste. Meanwhile, prepare the salad. Slice the fennel bulbs, the onion, the oranges and the black olives. Place the ingredients in a bowl and toss. Serve the fish on top of the salad and drizzle the remaining olive oil on top of everything.

GREEK SALAD

Ingredients
- *100 grams of Romaine lettuce*
- *1/2 red onion, tendered in warm water*
- *6 black olives*
- *200 grams of tomatoes*
- *200 grams of cucumber*
- *90 grams of feta cheese*
- *2 teaspoons of olive oil*
- *Oregano or basil*
- *1/2 squeezed lemon*
- *Salt and black pepper according to taste*

Preparation Cut all the ingredients into cubes, except for the onion, which should be thinly sliced. In a large salad bowl, combine the Romaine lettuce, onion, black olives, tomatoes, cucumber and feta cheese. Whisk together the olive oil, oregano/basil, lemon juice, salt and black pepper. Toss and serve.

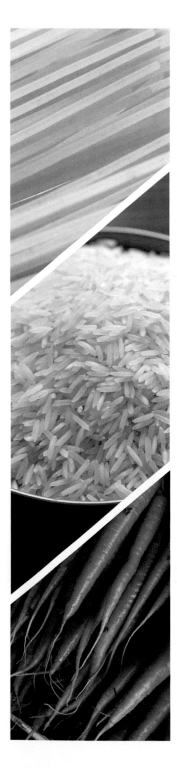

SPAGHETTI BOLOGNESE

Ingredients
- 2 tablespoons olive oil
- 1/2 white onion, chopped
- 1 carrot, chopped
- 2 celery legs, chopped
- 75 grams of lean mincemeat
- 1 glass of red wine
- 400 grams of tomatoes
- 100 grams of brown spaghetti
- Parmesan cheese, grated

Preparation In a large saucepan mix olive oil and two tablespoons of water. Over medium heat cook the onion until soft and brown. Stir in carrot and celery and cook until tender. When the vegetables are cooked, increase heat to medium heat, add meat and cook for 4 minutes until it has barely browned, tossing frequently with fork to break up clumps. Add the glass of wine. Boil rapidly for about 5 minutes until liquid has reduced slightly. Add the tomatoes, thinly diced and keep tossing until they start melting. Simmer, covered for 45 minutes, stirring occasionally. Meanwhile, in large saucepan, cook the spaghetti according to package directions and drain. Serve sauce immediately over hot spaghetti. And dust with a generous amount of grated Parmesan cheese.

FISH WITH RICE AND VEGETABLES

Ingredients
- 4 teaspoons of parsley, finely chopped
- 2 or 3 hot chilli peppers, finely chopped
- 2 or 3 cloves of minced garlic
- Salt and pepper to taste
- 150-180 grams of white fish in fillets
- 2 tablespoons of olive oil
- 2 onions, chopped
- 300 grams of tomatoes, finely chopped
- 3 carrots, sliced
- 1/4 head of cabbage, cut into wedges
- 1/2 eggplant, cubed
- 60 grams of rice
- Salt and pepper to taste

Preparation Mix the chopped parsley, chilli peppers, garlic, salt and pepper and cover the fillets with it. Heat the oil in a large, deep pot over medium heat. Brown the fish on both

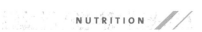

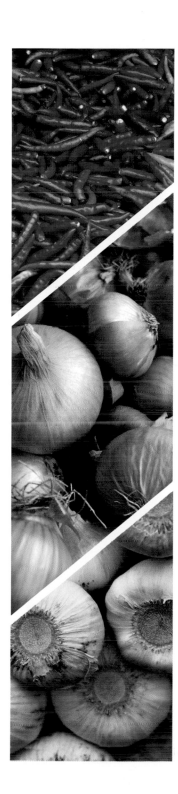

sides in the hot oil and remove to a plate. Add the chopped onions to the hot oil and sauté until cooked through and they are just beginning to brown (about 5 to 7 minutes). Stir in the tomatoes and let them melt, reducing the heat to low. Add some water then add the carrots, cabbage and eggplant and simmer over low heat for 35 minutes, or until the vegetables are cooked but not tender. Add the browned fish and simmer for another 15 minutes or so. Remove the fish and vegetables and about 1 cup of the broth to a platter, cover and set in a warm oven. Strain the remaining broth, discarding the solids. Add enough water to the broth to make 4 cups and return to heat. Bring the broth to a boil, stir in the rice and season with salt and pepper. Reduce heat to medium-low, cover and simmer for 20 minutes, or until the rice is cooked through and tender. Serve the fish over the rice, with vegetables around it.

Variations You can use whole fish or fish fillets. Any firm white-fleshed fish works well. Try this with snails (the best low GI meat you can find). Most vegetables work with this dish: try cassava, potatoes, green beans, zucchini, runner beans or peppers.

CHICKEN NOODLE SOUP

Ingredients
- *1 chicken, whole with skin (best is the corn-fed chicken)*
- *1 onion, roughly chopped*
- *1 celery leg, cut in half*
- *Salt and pepper to taste*
- *1 tablespoon of miso paste*
- *Piece of ginger root*
- *100 grams of rice noodles*
- *1 tablespoon minced garlic*
- *2 teaspoons finely chopped fresh parsley leaves or coriander*
- *1 lime*

Preparation Put the chicken, cut into pieces, the onion and the celery, in a large pan of cold water, add salt and pepper and bring to boil. Let it cook covered for about 1 hour. Then take the chicken out and choose the right amount of stock you need (depends if you are by yourself or feeding others), filter the fat out and put it in a smaller pan. Add the miso paste and two slices of ginger root to the stock and let it boil for 5 minutes. Add the noodles and let them cook for about 4 minutes. Take off the fire and serve in a broth bowl with 90 grams of the skinned chicken meat. Sprinkle with coriander or parsley and a squeeze of lime.

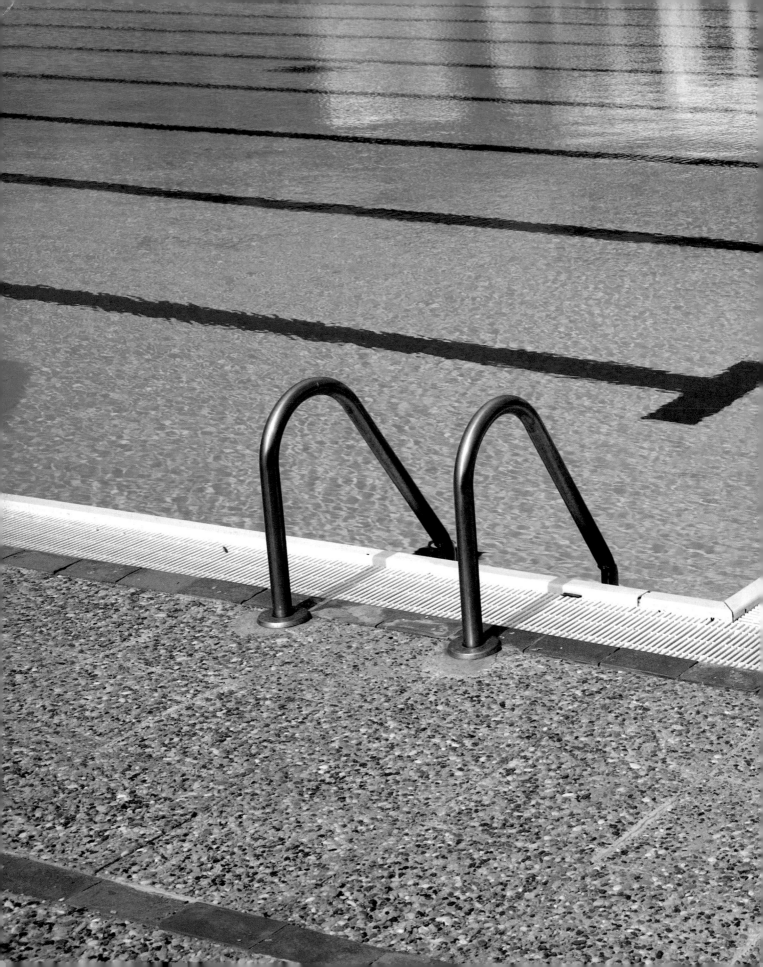

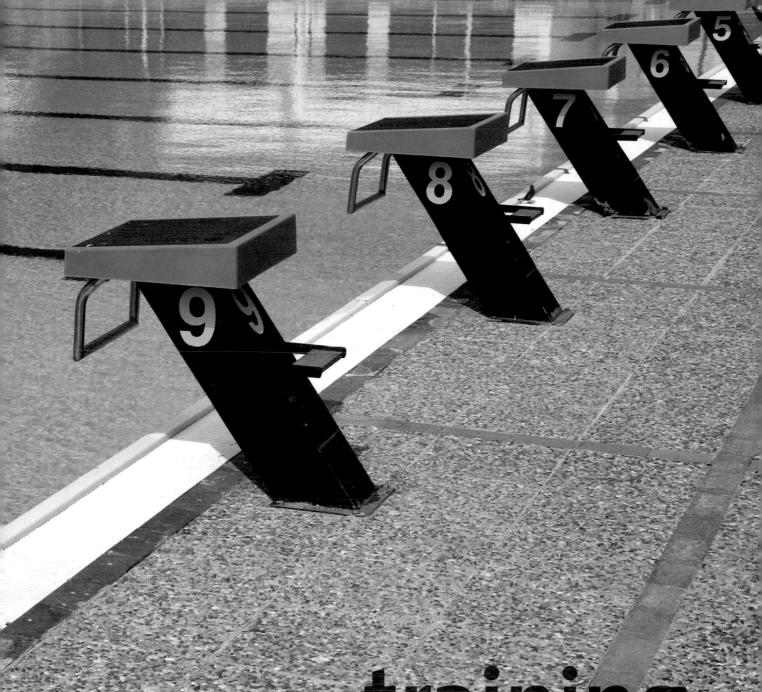

training programmes

// PLANNING // PREPARING // READY TO RACE

The basics

When developing a training programme you need to consider a number of things to make sure that it is going to be successful and allow you to achieve your goals. A training programme is a plan devised to ensure that you are able to swim at your peak level by the time you get to the day of your race.

There will be different phases during the training, which are vital in ensuring that you are ready to race. The training usually starts out less specific to the overall training goal and as you move through each phase the training becomes more specific to the race requirements. This is because it is important to have a solid training base to build on for future success. All training must lead to a goal otherwise your motivation can drop and improvements may slow down.

You need to first of all decide the following:

Why am I training?

You have to decide whether you are training for a specific competition, to improve your swimming technical ability or for fitness. If you plan to swim competitively then a training programme is vital to your success in the sport.

What am I training for?

Decide which type of event you are working towards (eg do you want to compete in sprint events such as 25m, 50m, 100m and 200m races, middle distance races such as 400m, or do you want to improve your distance swimming such as 800m, 1500m or 30/60 minute time trials?) Different events require different types of training. If you aren't training the right areas you will not improve at the speed you want to. You may decide you want to improve all the different areas of your swimming so you will have to get a good balance of sprint, aerobic and anaerobic training in your programme.

What do I want to achieve?

Is there a specific race you are training for? And if so when is it and how long do you have? If you have a specific race then you will need to plan your programme so that you can be at your peak for that race.

If you are trying to improve your ability and there is no set time frame you will want to be testing yourself to make sure that your training is doing what it is supposed to do. If you wish to improve your distance swimming then you will need to test your distance swimming ability at different stages throughout your training programme to ensure progression is occurring. If you find it isn't then you may need to evaluate your training programme and make suitable changes to ensure that steady progression occurs.

Things to remember

As with all training programmes you may find that during some sessions in the programme you aren't as good or as fast as you may have been in previous sessions. This does not mean that you should panic and change the programme; it may just mean that you have been working very hard and your body is tired. You should evaluate your training only at the end of each training cycle.

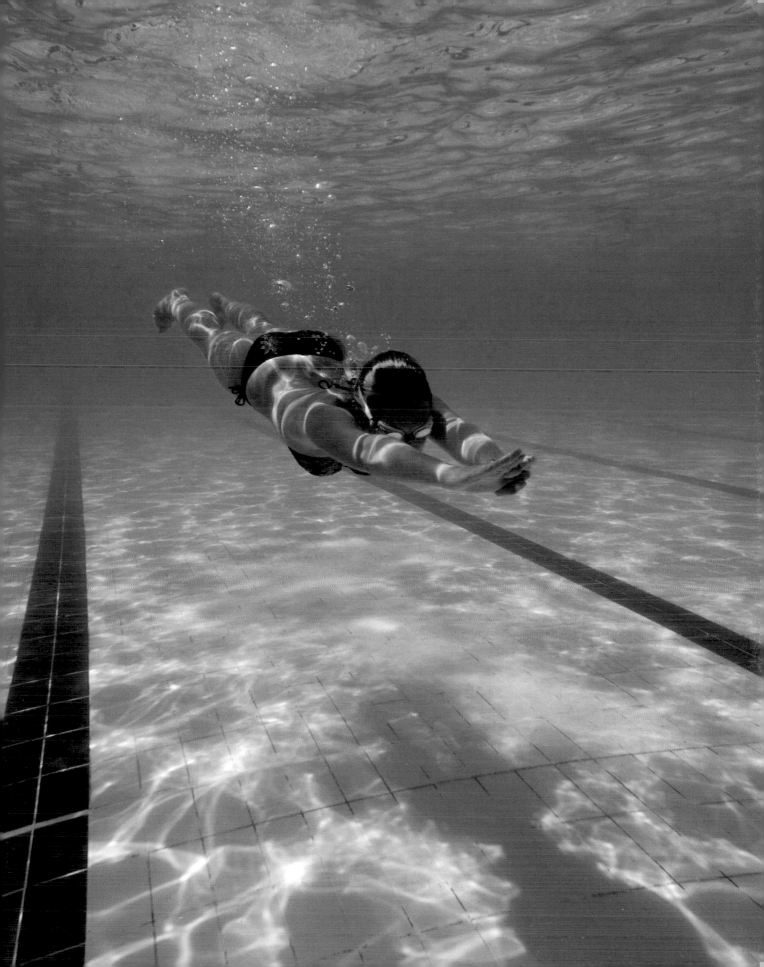

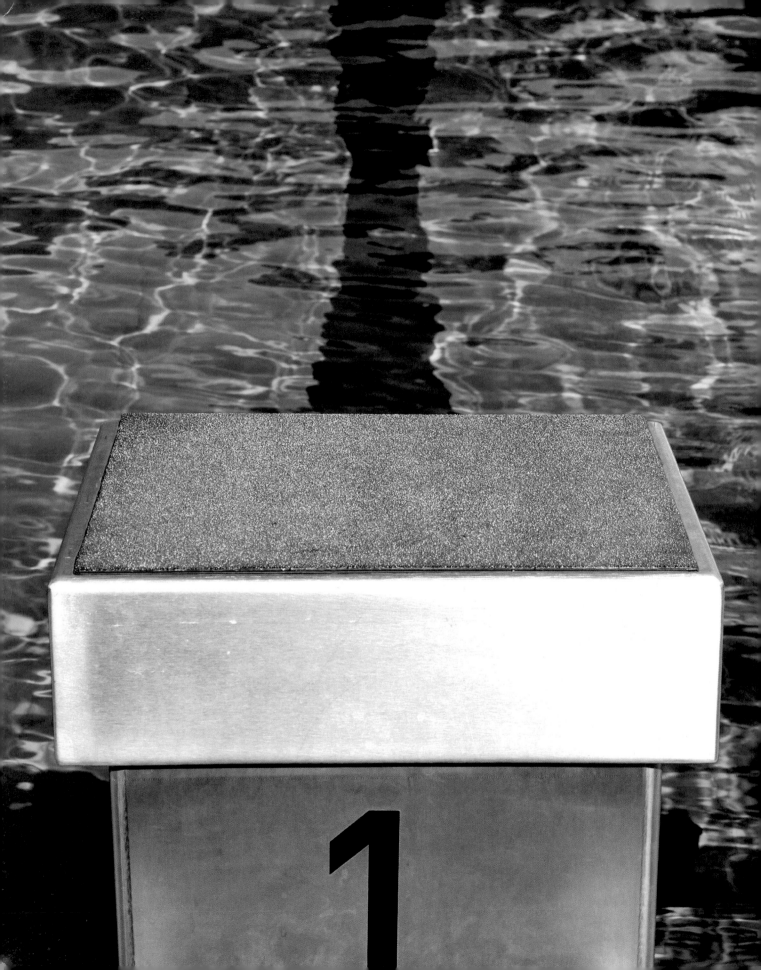

Planning your training

Periodization

Periodization is the breakdown of your training season or time frame into smaller manageable chunks where you may decide to focus on specific aspects of your swimming. Each phase of training will focus on improving an area of fitness while maintaining other areas of your performance at the same time.

The swimming season can be broken down into mesocycles, which last between six and 20 weeks. There will be a specific focus for each mesocycle, such as improving aerobic fitness and stroke technique, while at the same time maintaining sprint speed and threshold speed.

Within each mesocycle there is a microcycle, which refers to a smaller period (usually seven days). The microcycle contains a lot more detail and will specify exactly what training you will do each week during each session.

Depending on what your overall goal is – whether it is sprint swimming, middle-distance swimming or distance swimming, each mesocycle will be different, which is why it is so important to establish your goal clearly.

Tapering

Tapering is when you slowly reduce your training as the race approaches. If the training has been done in the weeks leading up to the race then your body will be ready and tuned, so extra hard training in the last few days will simply make you tired.

Tapering will be different for each and every swimmer but it is a crucial part of the training process because this is where you start to get physically and mentally ready to race and perform at your best.

The taper should reduce the overall amount of physical stress on your body, which will allow you to feel fresher and better prepared once you get to the race. Usually the overall training volume decreases while the workload stays fairly high.

A taper can be between two to five weeks long. During this phase you should ensure you are swimming large parts of your training in the stroke you intend to compete in and work on sets around the distance you intend to race at. In other words, in the last few weeks start to concentrate more and more on what you will be doing in the race. This can be either straight swims or broken swims (eg for 200m backstroke swimming you can do

200m backstroke sets in training or do broken swims such as 50-100-50 with short rests between each swim).

During the taper phase a lot of race preparation sets should also take place where you may work on a certain skill for the race such as underwater kicking or dives and turns. During this phase you should also take every precaution to limit stress on your body and eat and drink properly to ensure you stay healthy throughout the critical period. You have trained hard for many weeks so make sure you get it right in the critical last few weeks before race day.

Training zones

Training zone	Description	Details
EN-1	**Basic Endurance** This is the training zone used the most due to its lower intensity and the ability of swimmers to swim large volumes at this intensity without fatigue. It improves sub-maximal cardiovascular efficiency, which helps transport oxygen to working muscles. As the season progresses and your ability improves you will be able to swim EN-1 training sets at greater speed due to your increased fitness.	• Set lengths: minimum of 20 minutes and can be as long as time allows. • Rest intervals: 5-30 seconds. • Repeats: 50m+ can be used, as can different strokes. • Low-medium intensity.
EN-2	**Threshold Endurance** Used to build aerobic capacity without completely exhausting the energy system. It will also help improve lactate removal.	• Set length: 20-60 minutes. • Rest: 10-30 seconds. • Repeats: 50-400m. • Medium intensity.
EN-3	**Overload Endurance** Increases the maximal oxygen consumption. Increases the number of capillaries around the muscles. Increases the rate of lactate removal. Increases the buffering capacity of the muscle fibres.	• Set length: 20-45 minutes. • Rest: 5-30 seconds for 50/100s. 15-60 seconds for 200/400s and 30 seconds to 2 minutes for 800m+. • Repeats: any distance • High intensity

Training zone	Description	Details
SP-1	**Lactate Tolerance** Increases muscle buffering capacity. Improves your ability to maintain technique while swimming at high intensities with high levels of muscle acidosis. Improves blood lactate removal.	• Set length: 300-800m. • Rest: 1-4 minutes. • Repeats: 25-150m. • High intensity—maximum effort
SP-2	**Lactate Production** Short sprints at near maximum speed to help improve anaerobic power. Increases the amount of anaerobic metabolism. Increases maximum sprinting speed. Increases muscle buffering capacity. The difference between lactate tolerance and production is that production sets allow recovery swims to remove lactate before each repeat whereas tolerance sets make you swim with the lactate still present in your muscle.	• Set length: 300-600m. • Rest: 1-3 minutes of active recovery for 25m sprints and 3-5 minutes of active recovery for 50m repeats. • Repeats: 25-50m repeats are ideal. • Maximum effort, trying to get as close to personal best times.
RP	**Race Pace** As fast or faster than race pace, sometimes with the use of paddles or fins. Best done when you are fresh. Improves power and explosive strength in the water. Opportunity to practice swimming at race pace including fast starts/turns and stroke rates.	• Set length: 100-600m. • Rest: 1-6 minutes of active or passive recovery. • Repeats: dives, turns, 10m-25m sprints. • Maximum intensity

Planning for sprints

To improve your swimming over shorter distances such as 50m and 100m events and to some extent 200m events you will need to have a different training programme to those who wish to improve their distance swimming. The 50m events rely on the body to supply energy anaerobically, which means without the presence of oxygen for the majority of the race. Between 60-80 per cent of a 50m swim will be anaerobic depending on the fitness of the swimmer.

The 100m events still rely on the body to supply energy anaerobically for a large part of the race (up to 55 per cent) but the aerobic system will also have to supply energy for a substantial part of the race due to the duration of the swim. The 200m events, like 100m, will use both aerobic and anaerobic energy systems to supply energy for the race, which can be anything from 35-45 per cent of the race being swum anaerobically and the rest aerobically. The percentage being swum anaerobically will differ between each swimmer depending on fitness level, training background and genetic make-up

To be successful in sprinting you need to possess a high level of anaerobic metabolism and have the ability to swim quickly with high levels of lactate in your blood while still maintaining a good aerobic capacity.

Mesocycle 1 (8-14 weeks)

Each microcycle should include...

- Every session should contain some Basic Endurance (EN-1).
- You should try to do two Threshold Endurance (EN-2) sets each week.
- If you intend to swim 200m events then you should get one or two Overload Endurance (EN-3) sets in each week.
- Each week try to complete three-five Lactate Tolerance (SP-1) sets, which help the body buffer lactic acid when racing.

- You also need to get one Lactate Production (SP-2) set in each week.
- Include short sprint sets (RP) during each session.

You will sometimes be working more than one training zone in each session.

Example training week

Mon	*EN-1 + EN-2 + SP-1 + RP*
Tue	*EN-1 + EN-3 + SP-1 + RP*
Wed	*EN-1 + SP-2 + RP*
Thur	*Rest*
Fri	*EN-1 + EN-2 + SP-1 + RP*
Sat	*EN-1 + SP-1 + RP*
Sun	*Rest*

Mesocycle 2 (8-12 weeks)

Each microcycle should include...

- Basic Endurance (EN-1) training should be included in four-five sessions per week.
- You should try to do two Threshold Endurance (EN-2) sets each week.
- If you intend to swim 200m events then you should get one or two Overload Endurance (EN-3) sets in each week.
- Each week try to complete

three-five Lactate Tolerance (SP-1) sets, which help your body buffer lactic acid when racing.

- Include one big Lactate Production (SP-2) set in each week.
- Include short sprint sets (RP) during each session.

You will sometimes be working more than one training zone in each session.

Example training week

Mon	EN-1 + EN-2 + SP-1 + RP
Tue	EN-1 + EN-3 + SP-1 + RP
Wed	EN-1 + SP-2 + RP
Thur	Rest
Fri	EN-1 + EN-2 + SP-1 + RP
Sat	EN-3 + SP-1 + RP
Sun	Rest

Mesocycle 3 (4-6 weeks)

Each microcycle should include...

- Basic Endurance (EN-1) training should be included in four-five sessions per week.
- You should try to do one Threshold Endurance (EN-2) set each week.
- If you intend to swim 200m events then you should get one or two Overload Endurance (EN-3) sets in each week.
- Each week try to complete

three-five Lactate Tolerance (SP-1) sets, which help your body buffer lactic acid when racing.

- Include one big Lactate Production (SP-2) set in each week.
- Include short sprint (RP) sets during each session.

You will sometimes be working more than one training zone in each session.

Example training week

Mon	EN-1 + EN-2 + SP-1 + RP
Tue	EN-1 + EN-3 + SP-2 + RP
Wed	EN-1 + SP-2 + RP
Thur	Rest
Fri	EN-1 + SP-1 + RP
Sat	EN-3 + SP-1 + RP
Sun	Rest

Towards the end of mesocycle 3 you will be approaching your peak physical condition. As you lead up towards the race or time trial you should start to taper one-two weeks out by reducing the overall training volume, which allows your body more time to recover while not allowing the energy systems to start to reduce. If the taper is too long then the effects of all your hard work and training will be lost as your energy systems will start to show signs of reversibility.

Planning for middle distance

The demands of middle distance swimming are very different to sprint events as the body relies a lot more on the aerobic energy system and a lot less on the anaerobic system. Some 65-75 per cent of the swim will be swum aerobically and therefore the make-up of the training plan will be focusing more on building a strong aerobic base and a high aerobic threshold.

Middle-distance swimming covers 400m events but many middle-distance swimmers also compete at 200m and 800m.

The first two thirds of the training plan should focus on improving your aerobic capacity while maintaining other areas such as sprint speed and anaerobic threshold speed. It is not uncommon for other areas to slightly reduce due to the large amounts of aerobic training. During the final third of the training plan you should aim to maintain the large aerobic capacity while increasing the buffering capacity and anaerobic power.

Mesocycle 1 (8-16 weeks)

Each microcycle should include...

- Basic Endurance (EN-1) training should be included in every training session.
- Two-three Threshold Endurance (EN-2) sets should be included each week.
- One Overload Endurance (EN-3) set should be scheduled each week.
- Three-four Lactate Tolerance (SP-1) sets should be worked into each week.
- One major Lactate Production (SP-2) session should be scheduled each week

You will sometimes be working more than one training zone in each session.

Example training week

Mon	EN-1 + EN-2 + SP-2
Tue	EN-1 + EN-3
Wed	EN-1 + EN-2 + SP-1
Thur	Rest
Fri	EN-1 + SP-1
Sat	EN-1 + EN-2 + SP-1
Sun	EN-1 + SP-1

Mesocycle 2 (8-12 weeks)

Each microcycle should include...

- Basic Endurance (EN-1) training should be included in three-five sessions per week.
- One-two Threshold Endurance (EN-2) sets should be included each week.
- Two-three Overload Endurance (EN-3) sets should be scheduled each week.

- Three-four Lactate Tolerance (SP-1) sets should be worked into each week.
- One Race Pace (RP) session should be scheduled each week.

You will sometimes be working more than one training zone in each session.

Example training week

Mon	EN-1 + EN-2 + SP-1
Tue	EN-3 + SP-1
Wed	EN-1 + EN-3
Thur	Rest
Fri	EN-1 + EN-2 + SP-1
Sat	EN-1 + SP-1 + RP
Sun	Rest

Mesocycle 3 (4-6 weeks)

Each microcycle should include...

- Basic Endurance (EN-1) training should be included in three-four sessions per week.
- One Threshold Endurance (EN-2) set should be included each week.
- Two-three Overload Endurance (EN-3) set should be scheduled each week. The set distances should be shorter than in the previous cycle.

- Three-four Lactate Production (SP-1) sets should be worked into each week
- One Race Pace (RP) session should be scheduled each week.

You will sometimes be working more than one training zone in each session.

Example training week

Mon	EN-1 + EN-2 + SP-1 + RP
Tue	EN-1 + EN-3 + SP-2 + RP
Wed	EN-1 + SP-2 + RP
Thur	Rest
Fri	EN-1 + EN-3 SP-1 + RP
Sat	EN-3 + SP-1 + RP
Sun	Rest

Towards the end of mesocycle 3 you will be approaching your peak physical condition. As you lead up towards the race or time trial you should start to taper one-two weeks out by reducing the overall training volume, which allows your body more time to recover while not allowing the energy systems to start to reduce. If the taper is too long then the effects of all your hard work and training will be lost as your energy systems will start to show signs of reversibility.

Planning for long distance

Distance swimmers compete in the 800m and the 1500m but may also swim down to 400m events. Distance events will use the aerobic energy system to supply energy for the majority of the race (70-90 per cent) and therefore it is important that the large majority of training is aimed at improving your aerobic energy system.

Distance swimmers require a higher VO2 max and anaerobic threshold than swimmers who train for shorter events but will also have a lower ability when it comes to sprinting.

Mesocycle 1 (8-16 weeks)

Each microcycle should include...

- Basic Endurance (EN-1) training should be included in every training session.
- One-two Threshold Endurance (EN-2) sets should be included each week.
- Overload Endurance (EN-3) will be achieved by descending basic Threshold Endurance (EN-2) sets.
- Three-four Lactate Tolerance (SP-1) sets should be worked into each week.

You will sometimes be working more than one training zone in each session.

Example training week

Mon	*EN-1 + EN-2*
Tue	*EN-1 + SP-1*
Wed	*EN-1 + EN-2 + SP-1*
Thur	*Rest*
Fri	*EN-1 + SP-1*
Sat	*EN-1 + SP-1*
Sun	*Rest*

Mesocycle 2 (8-12 weeks)

Each microcycle should include...

- Basic Endurance (EN-1) training should be included in every training session.
- Two-three Threshold Endurance (EN-2) sets should be included each week.
- One-two Overload Endurance (EN-3) sets should be included each week.

- Two-three Lactate Tolerance (SP-1) sets should be worked into each week.

You will sometimes be working more than one training zone in each session.

Example training week

Mon	*EN-1 + EN-2*
Tue	*EN-1 + EN-3 + SP-1*
Wed	*EN-1 + EN-2 + SP-1*
Thur	*Rest*
Fri	*EN-1 + SP-1*
Sat	*EN-1 + SP-1*
Sun	*EN-1 + EN-3*

Mesocycle 3 (4-6 weeks)

Each microcycle should include...

- Basic Endurance (EN-1) training should be included in every training session. During mesocycle 3 the weekly total volume should start to be reduced by about a third.
- One-two Threshold Endurance (EN-2) sets should be included each week.

- Two Overload Endurance (EN-3) sets should be included each week.
- Three-four Lactate Tolerance (SP-1) sets should be worked into each week.

You will sometimes be working more than one training zone in each session.

Example training week

Mon	*EN-1 + SP-1 + EN-3*
Tue	*EN-1 + EN-2*
Wed	*EN-1 + SP-1*
Thur	*EN-1 + SP-1 + EN-3*
Fri	*EN-1 + EN-2*
Sat	*EN-1 + SP-1*
Sun	*Rest*

Towards the end of mesocycle 3 you will be approaching your peak physical condition. As you lead up towards the race or time trial you should start to taper one-two weeks out by reducing the overall training volume, which allows your body more time to recover while not allowing your energy systems to start to reduce. If the taper is too long then the effects of all your hard work and training will be lost as the energy systems will start to show signs of reversibility.

Example training sets

Training sets may require the use of equipment such as kick boards and pull buoys to help focus on specific areas of the stroke. Pull sets will focus on improving the arm stroke efficiency whilst kick sets will focus on warming up and improving leg kick. When kick and pull are used in warm-ups it is to help specifically warm up the specific area. Pull sets can also be used to help correct issues with arm stroke. By taking your legs out of the equation with pull buoy you can focus purely on improving your arm stroke.

Where sets require you to 'descend' it will mean that you have to get quicker on each rep. For example, if you are descending 6 x 100m freestyle you should be aiming to make each one a little bit quicker. You should be descending the time it takes you to swim each 100m.

Warm ups
- 800m mixed stroke.
- 4 x 200m (1 swim, 1 kick, 1 pull, 1 swim). Kick is with a kickboard and pull will be done with a pull buoy.
- 400m swim FC, 300m no FC swim, 200m FC, 100m no FC swim.
- 400m swim, 4 x 100 pull (with pull buoy), 4 x 50m kick (With kickboard).
- 8 x 100m (2 x 1 swim, 1 kick, 1 drill, 1 x IM).

Cool downs
- 200m–1000m mixed with swim, kick and pull.
- 5 x 100m, reducing speed each 100m.
- 2 x 300m, 1 x kick, 1 x swim.

EN-1 (Basic Endurance)
- FC set: 2-3 x (400m FC, 2 x 200m FC, 4 x 100m FC) All with 20 seconds rest between reps.
- FC set: 10 x 100m FC with 20 seconds between each 100m, 10 x 75m FC pull with 15 seconds rest between each 75m, 10 x 50m FC kick with 10 seconds rest between each 50m.
- IM set: 400m FC, 4 x 100m IM, 300m BS, 4 x 100m IM, 200m BK, 4 x 100m IM, 100m butterfly, 4 x 100m IM: All with 20 seconds rest between each rep.
- 2 x 200m (100m BF and 100m BK), 2 x 200m (100m BK and 100m BS), 200m (100m BS and 100m FC), 200 IM) All with 15 seconds rest between reps.

EN-2 (Threshold Endurance)
Threshold Endurance sets should be swam at 10-20 beats below your maximum heart rate. They should also have a perceived exertion of 15-16 on a scale of 1-20.
- 8 x 200m FC or your number one stroke.

- 2-4 x (2 x 200m and 1 x 100m) Increase your swim speed each round.
- 50m, 100m, 150m, 200m, 250m, 300m, 350m, 400m with 20-30 seconds rest between each rep.
- 4 x (4 x 100m). Descend 1-4 with 15 seconds rest between reps.

EN-3 (Overload Endurance)
Heart rate should stay close to maximum during Overload Endurance sets. Perceived exertion of 17-20 out of 20 is about right.
- 20-40 x 50m, with 15 seconds rest between each rep.
- 15-20 x 100m, with 10-30 seconds rest between each rep.
- 3 x 400m at best effort with one minute rest between each rep.
- 400m IM: one minute rest, 3 x 200m IM: 30 seconds rest, 4 x 100m IM with 15 seconds rest between each rep.

SP-1 (Lactate Tolerance)
- 4-6 x 100m with three minutes rest between each rep. Swims should be at best effort.
- 3 x 200m FC or your number one stroke off an eight-minute going time.
- 12 x 25m sprint with 30 seconds rest between each rep.
- 8 x 100m off a two-minute going time.

SP-2 (Lactate Production)

- 8 x 25m sprint off a two-minute going time.
- 4-8 x 50m sprint off five minutes. Actively recover between each rep.
- 3 x (4 x 25m your number one stroke sprint followed by 4 x 50m easy speed stroke drills)
- 4 x 50m maximum effort kick with three minutes rest between each rep.

RP (Race Pace)

All Race Pace training should be done when fresh so allow as much time to recover as needed between efforts to make sure they are all at your best effort.

- 8 x fast dives.
- 4 x 15m sprint.
- 4 x 10m sprints, 100m recovery, 4 x 15m sprints, 100m recovery, 4 x 25m sprints 200m recovery.
- 3 x (6 x 50m) As:
  1st 50m: 15m maximum, 35m easy.
  2nd 50m: 25m maximum, 25m easy.
  3rd 50m: fast dive, 50m easy.
  4th 50m: 35m maximum, 15m easy.
  5th 50m: fast dive, 50m easy.
  6th 50m: 50m maximum.

FC = freestyle, BK = backstroke, BF = butterfly, BS = breaststroke, IM = individual medley.

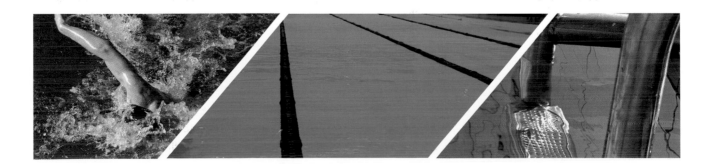

First published in 2011 by
New Holland Publishers (UK) Ltd
London • Cape Town • Sydney • Auckland
www.newhollandpublishers.com

Garfield House	80 McKenzie	Unit 1, 66	218 Lake Road
86–88 Edgware	Street	Gibbes Street,	Northcote
Road	Cape Town 8001	Chatswood	Auckland
London W2 2EA	South Africa	NSW 2067	New Zealand
United Kingdom		Australia	

A catalogue record for this book is available from the British Library.

ISBN 978 1 84773 781 6

This book has been produced for New Holland Publishers by
Chase My Snail Ltd
London • Cape Town

Project Manager: Daniel Ford
Designer: Darren Exell
Photo Editors: Darren Exell and Daniel Ford
Publisher: Guy Hobbs
Production: Marion Storz
Illustrators: Juliet Percival and James Berrangé
Proofreader: Timothy Shave

2 4 6 8 10 9 7 5 3 1

Reproduction by Pica Digital Pte Ltd, Singapore
Printed and bound in Malaysia by Times Offset (Malaysia) Sdn Bhd